The Complete Guide to the Menopause

Dr Annice Mukherjee is a hospital physician and endocrinologist with a medical career spanning almost 30 years. She trained as an undergraduate in Manchester and then worked in the South-East Thames region, based at King's College Hospital London, later returning to Manchester. She achieved a master's degree with King's College London and an MD thesis with the University of Manchester, which was based on quality of life in hormone diseases.

Dr Mukherjee took a consultant post at Salford Royal Hospital Foundation Trust, where she worked for 12 years. She specialises in general medicine and endocrinology with a career-long interest in complex medical illness, quality of life in hormone diseases and hormone problems in cancer survivors, including early menopause and other complex menopause issues, as well as managing chronic fatigue. She has supported thousands of women going through menopause to help them manage symptoms and safely improve their quality of life and overall health.

Dr Mukherjee prides herself on managing her patients in a holistic and innovative way. She always stresses that every single woman's menopause is different and their individual solutions will vary. She is uniquely and expertly placed to advise the modern woman to achieve a successful and healthy menopause.

Dr Mukherjee felt eternally grateful to have the knowledge that she had built up when she went through a breast cancer diagnosis and early menopause herself at the age of 41. Her knowledge enabled her to embrace and live life to the full, despite her health issues, and she wants to reproduce this positive experience for every woman going through menopause.

Dedicated to my father,
Amiya Pada Mukherjee

The Complete Guide to the Menopause

YOUR TOOLKIT TO TAKE CONTROL AND ACHIEVE LIFE-LONG HEALTH

Dr Annice Mukherjee

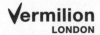

Vermilion
LONDON

Published in 2021 by Vermilion, an imprint of Ebury Publishing,
20 Vauxhall Bridge Road,
London SW1V 2SA

Vermilion is part of the Penguin Random House group of companies
whose addresses can be found at global.penguinrandomhouse.com

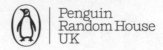

First published in the United Kingdom by Vermilion in 2021

www.penguin.co.uk

A CIP catalogue record for this book is available from
the British Library

ISBN 9781785043291

Typeset in 11/15 pt Sabon LT Std
by Integra Software Services Pvt. Ltd, Pondicherry

Printed and bound in Great Britain by Clays Ltd, Elcograf S.p.A.

The authorised representative in the EEA is Penguin Random House Ireland,
Morrison Chambers, 32 Nassau Street, Dublin D02 YH68.

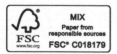

Penguin Random House is committed to a sustainable
future for our business, our readers and our planet.
This book is made from Forest Stewardship Council®
certified paper.

The information in this book has been compiled by way of general guidance in relation to the specific subjects addressed. It is not a substitute and not to be relied on for medical, healthcare, pharmaceutical or other professional advice on specific circumstances and in specific locations. Please consult your GP before changing, stopping or starting any medical treatment. So far as the author is aware the information given is correct and up to date as at July 2020. All names in cases studies have been changed. Practice, laws and regulations all change, and the reader should obtain up to date professional advice on any such issues. The author and publishers disclaim, as far as the law allows, any liability arising directly or indirectly from the use, or misuse, of the information contained in this book

Contents

Acknowledgements

Thank you to Lorna Stockwood, Jill and Ian Mukherjee, Sally Dynevor, Sally Harrison, Fairuz Awenat, Fiona Harrop, Alison Douglas, Helen Buckler, Anita Craven, Emma Persand, Julie Neville and my wonderful partner in life and husband, Simon Taggart, who all played an integral part, helping me, in different ways, to make this book happen.

Thank you also to all my very close and precious family and friends. I am not going to name you one by one, but I am truly grateful for your love, kindness and support.

Introduction

SO YOU ARE thinking about menopause. Perhaps you have noticed moments of feeling emotional for no particular reason. Maybe you broke out in a seemingly unexplained sweat during a work meeting. You may have woken in the night with your heart racing and could not get back to sleep. Such unexpected symptoms or sensations may have got you thinking that maybe this menopause business needs some exploring. Of course, you may be some way down the line from those symptoms and simply want to understand more about what menopause might mean for you.

Most women know they will experience menopause at some point but, historically, this has been a taboo subject, sometimes associated with negative connotations such as getting old and life slowing down. For the mature adult woman today, nothing could be further from the truth. For the majority, midlife has become enriched, fulfilled and busier than ever. We can now expect to have more adult life after menopause than any generation before us, because we are living longer. In light of this, our choices matter more than ever before.

Virtually all the new challenges facing you, as a woman going through menopause today, can be mitigated, resulting in empowerment and renewed vitality. Menopause mastery is a springboard for you to look and feel vibrant, and enjoy improved long-term quality of life. With the right approaches you can maintain a good level of fitness, keep energised, be more productive, thrive in the workplace for longer if you choose to and maintain stronger personal relationships. Modest lifestyle adjustments will facilitate many of these improvements and they will also reduce long-term health problems, resulting in an easier menopause transition and a more contented, healthy and fulfilled future.

The Complete Guide to the Menopause aims to provide essential information and furnish you with a practical toolkit to help you take control, feel empowered, successfully prepare for and manage your own menopause, and achieve lifelong health. The aim is to thrive, not just to survive. The solutions will include some universal codebreakers, effective for all, and some approaches that you can tailor to your individual circumstances. Each and every woman has a unique menopause experience. Symptoms are very varied and each of us will choose our own path depending on our circumstances. You may pass through with few symptoms or you may struggle with a multitude of problems. Regardless of symptoms, all women are united by a desire to maintain good health, well-being and self-confidence before, during and beyond menopause. In order to achieve this, you need to recognise and understand your own menopause transition and set about mastering it sooner rather than later.

The advice, strategies and information given cover almost every menopause scenario, enabling you to cherry-pick information according to your own individual needs. You may be interested in hormone therapies or seek lifestyle adjustments such as dietary guidance, improved sleep and stress management, among other things. This book celebrates your right to choose your own menopause path without judgement.

Part 1 will provide a general overview of menopause and decode it for you. This is important not only for those going through menopause, but those heading in that general direction, along with their partners and loved ones. It is really helpful for you and those close to you to understand the symptoms and how they may develop and progress as well as how they gradually settle down in time. Understanding the symptoms also helps you in implementing management strategies to overcome them. These strategies will be detailed in later chapters.

For those of you not yet experiencing menopause symptoms, it is important to keep perspective and not worry that you will experience every possible symptom. Many of you will be able to pass through menopause with modest lifestyle tweaks. But it is important to recognise that, for some of us, symptoms can escalate and become very disruptive. Medical support and treatment may be needed. For these reasons, I don't want to 'sugar-coat' the journey. I will be candid, but I will also provide solutions throughout the book. Everyone, including those worst-hit with menopause symptoms, can overcome any storms that menopause may produce and enjoy the anticyclone that you can achieve with the right actions and management going forward.

Part 2 involves empowering you with your own menopause toolkit. These chapters outline what you can do yourself without medication or the input of a doctor, as well as what can be done alongside these. They cover self-management approaches detailing how to conquer common menopause scenarios and symptoms that can hamper quality of life, with sustainable lifestyle adjustments that I describe as 'biohacks'. These should not be difficult to dovetail into your daily routine, but when implemented can be life-changing.

Part 3 provides information about management strategies that may be needed to support and complement lifestyle approaches. These chapters will help you to decipher which management approaches may be helpful in different symptom scenarios, including the benefits of HRT.

Part 4 discusses emerging considerations for menopause in the workplace and there is also a chapter for breast cancer survivors (an often excluded group when it comes to menopause discussion).

The book is structured in standalone sections, which can be read independently from one another, and does not need to be read sequentially. It can be used as a flexible tool to suit your own particular needs and interests. Each chapter is intended to be thought-provoking and to inspire you to make small, multidimensional changes and to enable you to be your own menopause expert. This will not only improve your personal menopause journey but also benefit those close to you.

So, let's set out to discover the best version of you, so you can live your best life. This is your opportunity to start the ball rolling to take control, be empowered and achieve lifelong health.

PART 1

Setting the Scene

CHAPTER 1

What is Menopause?

I N ORDER TO thrive in menopause, it is helpful for you to understand what it is. Menopause is a universal and natural biological process for all women, signifying the end of your fertile years. It is not an illness. The average age of menopause is 51 years. A small minority of us – 1 in 100 – will go through menopause before the age of 40 years, and approximately 1 in 1,000 women go through menopause under the age of 30.

If menopause has touched your life in any way you are not alone. Approximately 13 million women in the UK are peri- to postmenopausal – a third of the female population – and approximately 70–80 per cent of women experience symptoms.

WHY DOES MENOPAUSE OCCUR?

A girl is born with a lifetime store of eggs and the end of egg reserve is implicit in menopause. After birth, females do not make new eggs. At puberty the menstrual cycle kicks in, which, when balanced, results in rises and falls in oestrogen and progesterone in a very regulated pattern. This results in an egg being released every (or almost every) month. The ovaries also produce testosterone. No one knows with certainty for any individual the number of eggs remaining within the ovaries at any given time, when they will run out or when menopause will emerge. What is clear is that as a woman gets older, her egg reserve reduces. The number of eggs in the ovaries falls and the ability of the ovaries to produce hormones starts to decline. It is our current understanding that the decline in these hormones is integral to menopausal symptoms, which can appear well before periods stop altogether. At the time of menopause, virtually no eggs remain.

Although menopause is an entirely natural process, it does involve loss of function of the ovaries and the end of fertility, which is inevitable in every woman should she live long enough. It cannot currently be prevented. In this way, the menopause process is enigmatic and quite unique because no other organs or hormone glands (including the testes in males) are expected to naturally stop working in this way.

The timing of your menopause and the symptoms your body decides to give you are beyond your control. Nothing about menopause is your fault. You cannot stop menopause happening, but if you are armed with the right knowledge you can take action to lessen the impact of symptoms and optimise your menopause journey for the long haul.

Menopause symptoms are thought to be generated, at least in part, by deficiency of the ovarian hormones oestrogen, progesterone and testosterone. To understand how menopause unfolds let's briefly look at the different female hormone phases through life.

ADULT FEMALE HORMONE PHASES

Puberty

Puberty is a hormone transition, timed and controlled centrally in the brain's hypothalamus gland. During puberty, oestrogen levels steadily pulse in an upward direction with gradual development of adult female sexual characteristics, bone lengthening and maturing towards final height. This phase can cause a lot of hormone imbalance until the adult female hormone cycle stabilises. Puberty in girls is effectively the opposite of menopause, with low oestrogen at the start and fertile levels of hormones by the end.

Premenopause

After puberty, from her late teens, an adult woman with normal hormone production is described as being premenopausal. She is fertile and will usually have a monthly bleed. Several hormone imbalances can affect the periods in premenopausal women. The most common hormone imbalance in younger women is premenstrual tension (PMT), also described as premenstrual syndrome (PMS), which is linked to the drop in oestrogen and possibly changes in progesterone occurring in the latter stages of every monthly cycle. Many women will have experienced this to some degree. This natural drop in oestrogen can cause symptoms that are similar to menopause but, thankfully, are usually short-lived each month.

Pregnancy

Pregnancy results in a unique hormone phase all of its own, with oestrogen levels unparalleled by any other life situation. After pregnancy, a sudden free fall in oestrogen can result in symptoms such as baby blues, anxiety and sweats, which can mimic a mini-menopause. Oestrogen levels soon recover after pregnancy for most women and this post-pregnancy imbalance is usually short-lived and self-limiting.

Perimenopause

Perimenopause is effectively a transition period during which the hormone levels start to wax and wane. It most commonly occurs in a woman's mid- to late forties, but, as mentioned earlier, some women can enter perimenopause and progress into an early menopause in their early forties or even earlier, which is described as premature menopause if it occurs under the age of 40 years.

The ovaries can be quite erratic in the perimenopause. By erratic I mean that they can sometimes release an egg and sometimes not, and they can also produce surges of oestrogen (causing breast discomfort, migraines and heavy bleeding) followed by oestrogen crashes, which can be disruptive to well-being and induce some of the well-known menopause symptoms discussed in the next chapter.

During the perimenopause, the master hormone glands in the brain, which are called the hypothalamus and pituitary glands, sense that the ovaries are not working properly. The ovaries are usually receptive to two hormones produced by the pituitary gland: LH (luteinising hormone) and FSH (follicle-stimulating hormone). As perimenopause progresses, these hormones are upregulated, in essence to try to get the ovaries working again. As soon as the oestrogen rises in response to the LH and FSH rise, the latter tend to fall again.

So, in perimenopause hormone levels can be all over the place, which is why blood tests are not very useful and not necessary to diagnose perimenopause. Essentially, perimenopause is a hormone imbalance.

Perimenopause can last from a few months to several years. It's therefore not possible to say exactly when perimenopause is going to begin for each individual woman and it can also be difficult to pinpoint because the symptoms can be vague and non-specific. Early hormone fluctuations may be mild and go unnoticed. As hormone fluctuations progress, because the ovaries are not working properly, symptoms can start to become troublesome and periods can be affected and become irregular: they can be more or less frequent or simply erratic, and they can be lighter, heavier or of varying flow. Ultimately perimenopause gradually dovetails into full menopause.

Menopause

Menopause becomes established when the ovaries can no longer produce sustainable amounts of oestrogen. After menopause the LH and FSH from the pituitary gland remain permanently elevated as they sense there is no significant amount of oestrogen circulating. Oestrogen and progesterone remain undetectable after menopause. The ovaries also stop producing the male hormone testosterone. The adrenal glands continuously produce sex hormones after menopause, and small amounts of oestrogen and testosterone continue to be produced in fat cells.

DOES PREMENSTRUAL SYNDROME MORPH INTO PERIMENOPAUSE?

Science does not have a definitive answer to this yet but if you suffer from PMS, you may be more prone to symptoms during perimenopause. The two conditions can be difficult to distinguish.

Common symptoms in PMS include: mood swings, feeling upset, anxious or irritable, fatigue, sleep problems, bloating or tummy pain, breast soreness, headaches, skin breakouts, greasy hair and changes in appetite and sex drive. PMS is common; you are likely to recognise the symptoms to some degree. A rare form of PMS with the most severe symptoms is known as premenstrual dysphoric disorder (PMDD).

PMS can be relieved by lifestyle approaches, psychological treatments like cognitive behavioural therapy (CBT) and natural treatments such as starflower oil and agnus castus. Symptoms of PMS can also be relieved by using the combined contraceptive pill or using antidepressant medication. Perimenopause symptoms are relieved by oestrogen; however, oestrogen cannot be given alone unless you have had a hysterectomy. So, in most women who need hormone treatment for symptoms, progesterone needs to be given as well as oestrogen in combined HRT, to prevent womb thickening. Treatment of PMS-perimenopause benefits from medical advice from your doctor or hormone specialist. Certainly, getting PMS well controlled before perimenopause is likely to result in fewer symptoms in perimenopause.

Menopause is inevitable; it cannot currently be prevented. The age at which this occurs varies widely. The average age is 51 years, but it is not uncommon for women to still be having natural periods in their late fifties. Menopause may also occur prematurely, as mentioned above. Menopausal symptoms are often at their worst during the phase between peri- and postmenopause, but symptoms of menopause can span anything from 2 to 10 years and can also sometimes be almost non-existent. A few women will continue to have symptoms for more than 12 years. There is no clear explanation as to why the menopause experience is so variable, but symptom patterns can run in families so our genes may be at least in part to blame.

Postmenopause

Postmenopause is formally defined as the time after which a woman has experienced 12 consecutive months with no periods. For many women menopause symptoms may start to spontaneously improve from this stage, but if symptoms have been severe they can sometimes take longer to resolve and can continue despite menopause being complete.

KEY FACT

The take-home message for menopause stages is that perimenopause means early stages; menopause means fully-fledged; and postmenopause means all the time onwards from one year after periods stop.

TYPES OF MENOPAUSE

Most women will go through a natural menopause, but menopause can also result from medical conditions and there are interventions that can affect the timing of menopause.

OESTROGEN LEVELS IN THE DIFFERENT STAGES OF A WOMAN'S LIFE*

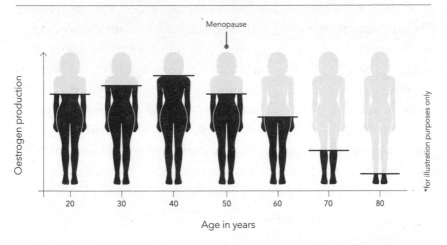

You will see that oestrogen levels can be very high in your forties. This can reflect surges and crashes in oestrogen as the ovaries misbehave and start to malfunction.

But fertility, which usually starts to reduce in this phase, can be unpredictable and sometimes fluctuating fertility in this stage can result in unexpected pregnancy.

Premature ovarian insufficiency (POI)

Also called premature menopause, POI is diagnosed if a woman's last natural period occurs before the age of 40 years. Menopause occurring under the age of 40 for any reason has some unique characteristics associated with it and so is considered quite differently in many ways from menopause occurring at an expected age. For example, women going through a very early menopause may have underlying medical conditions or genetic disorders that affect their ovaries. Examples include: damage to the ovaries due to autoimmune conditions producing antibodies that attack the ovaries; treatments that poison the ovaries, such as chemotherapy treatment for cancer; and genetic problems in which the ovaries don't function properly from the start. If you have POI you may also wish to have fertility treatment. The impact of oestrogen deficiency in women going through POI who are not treated can result in greater problems with bones and blood vessels in the longer term, because oestrogen is so important for these. Therefore women with POI are almost always treated with hormone therapies, at least until they reach a natural menopause age. They should be and are usually managed within specialist hormone clinics.

Early menopause

This is often used to describe women going into menopause between the ages of 40 and 45 years. While this is early, it is not classed as premature and is not generally treated differently from mainstream menopause.

Surgical menopause

Surgical menopause occurs if both the ovaries are removed. Younger women who have gynaecological problems and have both their ovaries removed may also be classified as POI, if this occurs under the age of 40 years. In this situation, hormone therapy is usually given until natural menopause age for its benefits to bone and heart health, as well as well-being. Thereafter, ongoing treatment is an individual choice.

If you have a hysterectomy due to gynaecological problems as a younger woman, you will more likely have one or both of your ovaries left in place. You will still produce oestrogen, progesterone and testosterone but you will not have periods. In this situation, it can be difficult for you to know when you are going through menopause as you won't have your period as a guide. If you have had a hysterectomy and had one or both ovaries left in place you may still be at greater risk of going into an early menopause, depending on your underlying gynaecological issues.

If you have a hysterectomy around the age of natural menopause, you will usually be advised to have a 'total hysterectomy', meaning both your ovaries and uterus are removed. The different surgical approach for pre-, peri- and postmenopause is because if you are premenopausal you are likely to have normal ovaries, so it is best to let your body produce its own natural hormones until you naturally go through menopause, rather than remove the ovaries and give you hormone replacement that you didn't necessarily need. If you are postmenopausal and need a hysterectomy your ovaries are no longer working, so they will usually be removed during your hysterectomy, as this causes no harm and eliminates any risk of ovarian cancer later.

Chemical menopause

You can have menopause 'induced' temporarily with hormone treatments that block the menstrual cycle altogether. This type of menopause induction is used to treat conditions such as endometriosis and other gynaecological problems. It is also quite commonly used for premenopausal breast cancer treatment if the cancer is oestrogen receptive. This type of treatment is not needed or used in women who have already gone through menopause. It aims to block oestrogen production from the ovaries for a period of time as part of treatment for the underlying condition. This type of menopause is generally temporary, so when the treatment stops, hormones normalise and periods resume. If the treatment is given when you are already perimenopausal then your ovaries would have been heading towards menopause anyway. In this situation chemical treatment may induce menopause permanently.

A quick recap

You go through several different hormone stages and changes during your life, and with each one your body changes. The timing and circumstances of hormone fluctuations and changes can be affected by our genes as well as health problems along the way. Each and every one of us will have a different experience in each of the hormone stages. The final hormone change is menopause, which all of us will experience at different times and in different ways.

Understanding what symptoms you might expect will help you to recognise that you may be entering menopause, which is the focus of the next chapter.

CHAPTER 2

Demystifying Symptoms

UNDERSTANDING THE SYMPTOMS of menopause is important, but you must remember that not everyone gets every symptom. Some women get none and for many women symptoms may be noticeable but mild. If you have not started with menopause yet you may still relate to some of the symptoms from your PMT symptoms during your monthly cycle. Understanding more about them should therefore be helpful as you will be forearmed that any new symptoms may indicate the start of menopause. Equally, if you are already in menopause, don't expect that if you have not had one of the symptoms described it will be inevitable. Women experience menopause in very different ways.

Most symptoms of menopause relate to oestrogen deficiency, but some are linked to low progesterone and testosterone. More recent research suggests that some brain hormones, secreted by the hypothalamus gland, may also play a major part in menopausal symptoms including hot flushes. In these studies, a novel medication (neurokinin 3 receptor antagonist), which could be safe for many women including those who cannot take HRT, is currently being trialled and they are showing very good results. This is exciting stuff but we need to watch this space as the treatment is not quite ready for the mainstream yet.

MENOPAUSE NOW

The years in a woman's life leading up to and during menopause today are often profoundly busy and complicated. Nowadays women in their forties to sixties may have challenging and demanding careers, be raising children, caring for ageing parents, have non-paid voluntary commitments that are demanding, among other challenges, and they may themselves be living with health issues or long-term conditions. These factors can all impact on the extent and severity of menopausal symptoms.

COMMON SYMPTOMS

I will keep reiterating that menopause is different for every woman, so there will be some symptoms that you may not relate to. Not every woman gets every symptom, thankfully!

KEY FACT

Approximately 70–80 per cent of all women will suffer from menopausal symptoms. The severity and duration of symptoms is very variable, usually ranging from two to ten years, with the average at seven years.

Menopause is famous for symptoms. Symptoms can occur before menopause shows up on blood tests. Even without any treatment, symptoms usually gradually and spontaneously improve over 2–10 years, once your periods stop and your body adjusts to the new status quo.

As I discuss symptoms, unless stated specifically, the symptoms you experience tend to persist from perimenopause and into full menopause and then usually start to lessen in postmenopause. The following list covers the most common symptoms that women may experience. However, it is quite possible that you have experienced a menopause symptom that is not included here. If so, you may have a rare symptom of menopause. Or perhaps the symptom is not related to your menopause at all!

Erratic periods

Some women can have erratic periods for years before they finally stop altogether, while for others the periods stop overnight. It is not uncommon to miss a few bleeds, think you are through, and then have a heavy downpour or two before they fizzle out again. This variation occurs because production of oestrogen by the ovaries usually fluctuates downwards rather than nosedives. Dips in oestrogen production can be followed by surges as the ovaries try to respond to feedback from the pituitary gland hormones LH and FSH (see page 10). When oestrogen levels are low, the lining of the uterus thins and bleeding becomes minimal. After an oestrogen surge, the womb lining can thicken considerably. It is the womb lining that sheds to produce the monthly period in fertile women. In perimenopause bleeding can be heavy and dysfunctional when the lining rapidly thickens in response to oestrogen surges and then sheds erratically. The heavy periods can also sometimes cause iron deficiency due to the blood loss.

Eventually oestrogen deficiency dominates, the womb lining becomes persistently thin and periods cease altogether. This can be a huge relief to women who have had heavy periods before menopause. Menopause and the end of periods can be liberating for women who have been in this situation in pre- and perimenopause.

Hot flushes and sweats

These are the symptoms most people identify with menopause. They are so important that I have dedicated Chapter 6 to them.

Every woman's experience will be different. Some women will have sweating episodes, day and night. Some will experience a heat or flushing sensation. Some women will not be bothered by the presence of sweats when they occur, but the 'drenching night sweats' scenario is unpleasant for many women and can disrupt sleep. Hot sweats and flushes are often followed by a sense of feeling the chills and can be accompanied by palpitations and anxiety. For most women the symptoms ease with time but the duration is unpredictable.

These symptoms are usually at their worst during the first year after the periods cease (in the year from menopause to postmenopause). The average duration of hot sweats is very variable but will last two years or fewer for about 80 per cent of women.

The cause of menopausal flushes and sweats has long been elusive. It is clear that the cause relates to hormone fluctuations, but the exact mechanism remains poorly understood. Some newly discovered brain hormones may hold the key to the cause and a potential cure for menopausal flushes and sweats (as mentioned earlier), and are currently the subject of intense study.

Sleep disruption

It is common to experience sleep problems during menopause, but sleep difficulty is frequently not only due to menopause. With busy schedules, positions of responsibility at home and at work, high levels of stress and little time for self-care or self-compassion, adult women today, and in particular women in their forties to sixties, have plenty of reasons to have disrupted sleep, even without the hormone changes in menopause. Nonetheless, menopause can bring another layer to sleep disruption at this stage in life.

As hormone levels decline during menopause many, but not all, women experience some degree of sleep disruption. Oestrogen does promote healthy sleep – it helps the body use serotonin and other neurochemicals that assist sleep. If oestrogen is low it is therefore important to address other factors that disrupt serotonin, such as chronic stress, poor diet and heavy chronic alcohol intake, among other factors. Serotonin depletion also negatively affects mood and can impact on melatonin – the circadian rhythm hormone that regulates the sleep cycle.

Natural progesterone is largely a sleep-promotor. Progesterone tends to promote a sense of calm, boosting relaxation and facilitating sleep. Progesterone increases production of GABA (gamma-aminobutyric acid), a neurotransmitter that helps sleep. Low progesterone can bring about anxiety and restlessness, and therefore trouble sleeping.

Other menopausal symptoms, like night sweats, palpitations and anxiety, can also contribute to disrupted sleep. For those who are troubled with sleep difficulties in menopause, there is lots of practical advice and prescriptive strategies about managing sleep problems in Chapter 7.

Changes in mood

Most women are aware that hormone fluctuations can affect mood and most will have experienced this within their fertile years during their normal monthly cycle. During each monthly cycle in premenopausal women, oestrogen levels climb and reach a peak around day 14 after bleeding starts, which coincides with ovulation. Thereafter levels decline and when they get to a low level at the end of the month bleeding is triggered. As the oestrogen level declines leading up to the period most women do not feel at their best in terms of well-being and mood because oestrogen is a feel-good hormone.

From perimenopause, fluctuating oestrogen can disrupt mood similarly, but a little more unpredictably, than it does during premenopause. Major mood problems such as severe depression are thankfully not very common in menopause, but it is likely that you will experience some mood changes. Symptoms including anxiety, irritability and mood swings are quite common. As with other menopausal symptoms, these usually gradually settle with time.

Low oestrogen can be a trigger for low mood, but there are many other factors that will dictate if a particular woman will suffer with mood problems, such as historic and ongoing stress, major life events, genetic factors and previous history of depression or trauma.

Being unpredictably and unexpectedly irritable can be upsetting, but these mood changes are usually temporary, often mild and not everyone will experience them. They are likely to be worse if you are stressed and under pressure. In these situations it is important for you to ensure that you apply self-care and understand that it's a phase that will pass. There are many actions you can take to smooth out moodiness, and I will discuss troubleshooting these symptoms in Chapters 9 and 15.

Joint and muscle aches

The effects of lower oestrogen levels, from the perimenopause onwards, can result in general aches and pains.

Muscle and joint aches often trigger an instinctive response to do less physical activity and movement. This is exactly the wrong response because exercise and movement strengthen muscles, tendons, ligaments and bone, and so exercise can actually counteract and balance the effect of low oestrogen on these tissues after menopause. Activity and movement will often improve aches and pain as long as the exercise is built up gradually (see Chapter 4).

Changes in body shape

Oestrogen and testosterone both influence metabolism. Loss of testosterone in men appears to cause greater effects than it does in women, but testosterone deficiency can contribute to issues in women after menopause too. As these hormone levels fall in menopause, the metabolic rate drops. This means it is easier to gain weight, but weight gain is multifactorial and HRT does not prevent it. Weight is also deposited more around the middle as we get older.

In the Western world, weight and body mass index (BMI), which is a calculation of weight in proportion to height, have been increasing in recent decades in all age groups. One report in August 2019 quoted that the rate of obesity had risen in adults in England from 15 per cent in 1993 to 29 per cent in 2017. Thirty-seven per cent of women in this cohort were found to have a normal BMI, 31 per cent were found to be overweight and 30 per cent obese.

Preventing weight gain and keeping weight at a stable level is a challenge for everyone in today's society, but it is doable, both before and through menopause, with the right information and guidance and a mindful approach to eating – more about this in Chapter 8.

MENOPAUSE NOW

Women reaching menopause today are more likely to be carrying excess weight compared with women going through menopause only a few decades ago. Many health issues occurring after menopause may be linked with weight increases, such as type 2 diabetes, which affects 6 per cent of the UK population and is more common with increasing age, and an underactive thyroid, which can affect up to 20 per cent of women over the age of 50. Keeping a healthy weight is important to reduce risks of many health conditions as you get older.

Skin, hair and nail changes

It is important not to blame menopause for everything to do with ageing. There are complex effects of ageing on skin, hair and nails that are not just all about oestrogen deficiency. Men don't have a male menopause but they still age! Data are inconclusive about whether HRT improves wrinkles in sun-exposed areas of skin, highlighting the likely contribution of other factors that predispose to skin ageing, hair thickness and nail quality. Sun damage from years or decades of excessive sun exposure, smoking, excess alcohol, poor diet and micronutrient deficiencies all contribute to your skin, hair and nail quality throughout adult life, as well as your integrated health. While hormone therapy may help with some aspects, it is not a panacea for ageing and it is not a substitute for keeping yourself healthy, inside and out, to reduce the effects of ageing.

Oestrogen is linked to melanin production in the skin, so when oestrogen levels fall, sun exposure can have different effects: the skin tends to tan less easily, more patchily and can burn and damage more easily, so you need to take more care with sun exposure and use plenty of sun protection to keep your skin healthy and reduce the effects of sun damage that increase skin ageing after menopause.

Oestrogen increases blood flow to the skin, increases skin collagen content and skin moisture, and maintains skin thickness. Dehydration can be a general common problem as we get older and this can also contribute to skin dehydration, so drinking plenty of water is a good counterbalance to dehydrated skin (see page 68).

Another skin symptom in menopause is an altered skin sensation called formication, which is itching that can feel like insects crawling over the skin. This can occur in a number of physical health issues, including diabetes, shingles, some infections and withdrawal from some medications including some antidepressants, and can sometimes occur in perimenopause and menopause. It is not very common, but when problematic during menopause it can be treated with antihistamines or with treatments used for hot flushes and sweats (see Chapter 6).

Oestrogen strengthens hair and nails. Decreasing levels of oestrogen and progesterone can affect hair and nail growth and quality. It is therefore important to pay attention to factors that can mitigate these effects, such as ensuring good levels of micronutrients that contribute to healthy hair and nails (see Chapter 5 for more on this).

Vaginal symptoms, loss of sex drive and bladder issues

As oestrogen levels fall in perimenopause there can be significant effects on the vagina. Like in other tissues, oestrogen increases blood flow to the vagina and hydrates it. The decline in oestrogen levels around menopause results in reduced blood flow to the lining of the vulva, vagina and cervix. The vaginal skin can become thinner and more vulnerable to infection and trauma. These changes may be described as vulvo-vaginal atrophy.

Symptoms of vaginal oestrogen deficiency around menopause most commonly include vaginal dryness, pain on intercourse, vulval and vaginal itching and discharge. The urinary tract can also be affected, leading to the need to pass urine more often, needing to pass urine during the night, urgency, pain on urinating and urinary incontinence. Recurrent urine infections occur in up to 20 per cent of postmenopausal women because of thinning of the lining of the bladder and urethra (bladder pipes) due to low oestrogen.

Vaginal symptoms can be hard to deal with during menopause. This is because they not only result in physical symptoms, but can negatively affect intimacy and sexual health, and can therefore impact on relationships. Psychological factors come into play when a woman has physical symptoms that can affect sexual function. This may result in intimacy and penetration being off-putting. These are described as 'psychosexual' factors.

A woman may resent herself or feel inadequate or frustrated that she doesn't want to have sex because of fear of pain, discomfort or due to lack of interest. On the other hand, she may feel resentment towards her partner for pressuring her into it. This can create a complex dynamic. If not addressed, this can add to strain on relationships and even result in relationship breakdown. Vaginal symptoms are therefore very important to acknowledge and address. Suffering in silence is not OK. Sweeping it under the carpet will not help. There are management strategies and treatments that can make a positive difference and this is a topic that needs greater public health attention. Treatment options and strategies to combat vaginal symptoms are discussed in Chapter 2.

Breast issues

Breast soreness related to perimenopause may feel different from the soreness you may have felt at other times in your life. Breast pain during perimenopause may feel like burning or soreness, or may be sharp, stabbing or throbbing. You may feel it in one breast or both breasts. Not all women experience breast discomfort in the same way. This can usually be relieved by taking evening primrose or starflower oil supplements (see page 172).

If you are worried about breast soreness it is always best to see your doctor and get checked out. It is helpful to get into a routine of checking your breasts at the same time every month. If you are having periods it is best to check just before your period. That way you get to know your own breasts and will notice a difference if a change occurs.

The following symptoms indicate that you need to see a doctor to get a detailed check:

- clear, yellow, bloody or pus-like discharge from the nipple
- increase in breast size
- redness of the breast
- changes in the appearance of the breast: lumps, swelling, dimpling, rash, nipple inversion
- fever
- chest pain

Brain fog

Menopause-related cognitive impairment, more commonly known as brain fog, is experienced by many women in perimenopause and menopause. Symptoms range from mild transient memory

KEY FACT

One in eight women in the UK is expected to develop breast cancer during her lifetime, and self-awareness is likely to aid early diagnosis. The earlier a breast cancer is picked up, the more successful and usually less aggressive the treatment. So it's important that you check your breasts regularly and see a doctor if you notice any changes.

issues to more severe working memory and attention issues, and difficulty focusing and learning new skills. These can be problematic in the workplace and may require some work adjustments to prevent them impacting on work roles (see Chapter 16).

The exact cause of menopause brain fog is not well understood and severity varies between individuals. Factors that may be present in menopause, such as micronutrient deficiencies, in particular B vitamins, zinc and iron deficiencies, chronic stress, pre-existing mood disorders, such as anxiety and depression, and thyroid problems, among other issues, can all impact on brain focus. Addressing these can make a positive difference to symptoms, and solutions will be covered in Part 2.

Memory function does improve gradually over time during menopause, even in women not treated with hormone therapy, which suggests that this symptom is not solely caused by low oestrogen, but relates more to the hormone fluctuations and changes during menopause, in a similar way to women who experience 'baby brain' when they have had a baby!

Headaches and migraines

Menopause can affect headaches in several ways. The effects will be different for every woman. Many premenopausal women experience severe headaches that appear to be linked to hormone changes. Migraines are a subtype of headache. These are typically the most debilitating of headaches. It was previously thought that migraines were always characterised by throbbing pain on one side of the head, nausea, sickness, sensitivity to light or sound, and visual auras. We now know that migraines can be experienced in many different ways and the condition is often now referred to as 'migraine spectrum disorder'. Many women experience migraine worsening on the pill and sometimes during pregnancy; situations where oestrogen levels are high.

For women who experience cyclical headaches and migraine symptoms in the premenopause, the symptoms may relate to hormone fluctuation and in particular oestrogen fluctuations. For these women, the progression of symptoms in menopause will depend on how their menopause progresses. For example, if a woman has a rapid progression through menopause and oestrogen deficiency occurs quickly, she may experience rapid relief of hormone-driven symptoms of headache and migraines. If the same woman experiences a fluctuating perimenopause with hormones going up and down for months or years, she may experience worsening of her hormone-driven headaches for a period of time until she reaches postmenopause.

Some women will continue to experience migraines after menopause is complete, but the majority of women will have some degree of remission or resolution of headaches and migraines after menopause. Any woman developing a new onset of progressive migraine-type headaches around menopause, when they did not suffer migraines before menopause, should be thoroughly assessed and investigated for other neurological causes of headache.

Fatigue

Fatigue can be triggered and driven by many different factors. In menopause, there are a multitude of potential triggers for fatigue, particularly for women in today's world. It is important for you to be aware that fatigue is quite widespread in the whole of society, not just in menopause. It is frequently fuelled by reversible factors and conquering fatigue is a great skill to boost well-being at any age.

Examples of factors that can trigger or worsen fatigue in menopause include: sleep disruption, anxiety, pain from headaches, muscles or joint pain, low mood, iron and other micronutrient deficiencies, along with stress, major life events and any other coexisting health issues that you have.

Some of these factors relate to the decline in hormones occurring in menopause. Some symptoms relate to collateral effects, like iron and other micronutrient deficiencies, while other symptoms are unrelated, independent problems that are fatigue triggers, which may happen to occur more often in women of menopausal age, such as relationship difficulties, stress relating to a care role, bereavements and health issues such as diabetes, thyroid problems, fibromyalgia and arthritis, among others.

Instinctive responses to fatigue can make it worse and the right approaches to reduce fatigue can be counter-intuitive. Many self-directed strategies can be applied to improve symptoms of fatigue (see Chapter 11).

A quick recap

Understanding that new symptoms may be due to menopause is helpful and important because you can seek prompt help from your doctor if they progress and become bothersome despite your best efforts with lifestyle approaches and self-management. There are many different treatments available for menopause symptoms and you should never feel that you have to suffer in silence. For most of us symptoms settle over time, so if your symptoms escalate and affect your quality of life it is better to seek help sooner rather than later to get your well-being back on track.

Now that we have explored the various symptoms of menopause, it's time to find a tailored, individual solution for you. Like solving a Rubik's cube, it can be easy when you know how!

CHAPTER 3

Taking Back Control

I F YOU SEEK help from a doctor about menopause symptoms you may well be given a prescription for an antidepressant, sleeping aid or painkiller, not because you want or need medication, but because trying to achieve a simplistic health solution with a prescription medication is engrained in our healthcare culture. In our current healthcare system, lifestyle approaches are not usually a central focus, and instead doctors or specialists will generally only look at one symptom and try to fix it. Often you will be prescribed a medication and this may have side effects, and the treatment offered may not address the underlying problem in a comprehensive and effective way. When simple treatments don't work, women are often simply reassured that there is nothing serious and symptoms are dismissed.

Menopause involves a complex array of symptoms arising as a result of differences in functioning in a large number of systems in the body, many of which are interconnected. The net result for you will also be influenced by the modern world environment, which is different from any time in history. You cannot therefore view menopause in a simplistic or linear way, and these intricacies help to explain why some women do not achieve well-being balance in menopause, sometimes even during treatment with HRT.

The idea of taking control of your well-being and improving your health is something that most women – and, indeed most adults on the planet – wish to achieve. It is very easy to judge, but it is clear to me that no one chooses to be overweight, inactive, stressed or exhausted! If you can figure out where things have changed for you, you can then fix the issues methodically and systematically. This is where my lifestyle toolkit comes in.

You will need a number of different 'tools' to fix each particular symptom or system. Many of those tools will be small measures and tweaks that in isolation do not seem significant, but a combination of these strategies will be so much more effective and sustainable than the single magic-bullet fix that we all sometimes wish for and that the Internet often falsely promises. These multi-faceted interventions will be different for each and every one of us. Your menopause lifestyle toolkit will be unique to you – one size does not fit all.

Small incremental lifestyle approaches that can alter your body's biology for the better and benefit your health and well-being are sometimes called 'biohacks'. Each chapter in Part 2 highlights important menopause concerns and provides tailored solutions for you to overcome them. When used in combination, this toolkit enables multiple small and relatively easy changes, or biohacks, to provide you with sustained, positive health and well-being benefits. The more systems that are positively balanced, the greater the health benefits.

I cannot resolve global wellness problems in one fell swoop. I can, however, provide a framework (a biohacking toolkit) to empower you to successfully sustain changes, which will make a positive difference to your quality of life and long-term health.

THE HOUSE OF MENOPAUSE

Lifestyle tweaks work because they are small changes in many systems of the body, rather than one big change. Putting all your eggs in one basket will rarely improve overall well-being in meno-pause because symptoms are so intricate and interconnected.

Imagine your menopause well-being is a house in winter with the central heating on, but all the windows have been opened so the heat (energy) is escaping. Each individual window losing energy represents each of the systems in the human body that contribute to your overall well-being and energy levels. If you close one window in the house, you can't expect the house to get warm when there are, perhaps, another 10 windows letting the energy and well-being out.

Say you identify the first open window as your sleep being disrupted and you assume that must be causing a lot of your problems. You sort out your sleep patterns, improve your sleep routine, relax before bedtime, stay off your phone – you do all the right things – and yet you still don't wake up feeling refreshed. In this situation, the instinctive response is to think the sleep changes you have made have not worked, so you abandon all your good efforts to improve sleep. You then reopen that (sleep) window and try to close another window instead – say focusing on diet or seeking medication.

The fact is that even if you sort out your sleep brilliantly using state-of-the-art measures that you know should be helpful, and

THE HOUSE OF MENOPAUSE:
HOW TO BOLSTER YOUR WELL-BEING

Depletes well-being ⟵----- Balance between energy ⟶ Preserves well-being
loss and preservation

· Stress
· Poor sleep
· Inactivity
· Boom/bust activity
· Erratic lifestyle
· Being chronically overburdened/ overwhelmed
· Pain
· Poor diet
· Micronutrient depletion
· Carrying excess weight
· Some pain and mood medications
· Using alcohol and smoking as coping strategies

· Stress management
· Good sleep routine
· 30 minutes of dedicated physical activity every day
· Avoiding boom/bust activity
· Regular lifestyle routine
· Being realistic about what you can achieve
· Healthy diet
· A–Z micronutrient optimisation
· Keeping a healthy stable weight
· Avoiding unhelpful medication
· Avoiding use of alcohol and smoking as coping strategies

31

indeed are needed, it may not be enough in isolation to improve your well-being. There are so many other factors at play in menopause that using a single linear approach will not deliver the reward of making you feel better.

For each and every woman going through menopause, some systems will be impacted more than others, just like different sized windows in a house have different energy loss impacts if left open. So, if you have been a lifelong insomniac, you may struggle with problematic sleep disruption and fatigue as menopause hits. If anxiety is your nemesis then that may trouble you in menopause and may be associated with symptoms such as palpitations or low mood. Similarly, for weight balance, muscle and joint aches and other issues, there are patterns of symptoms that can surface during menopause that may or may not have troubled you to some extent in your premenopausal years. These are like the different sized windows in your own house of menopause and many strategies are needed to rebalance well-being.

This house of menopause metaphor is about helping you to understand how to make your unique house energy efficient, 'one window at a time'. Make sure you close all the windows, or at least as many as possible, room by room. The solutions in the toolkit in Part 2 will help you to do this.

HOW TO SUCCEED WITH YOUR LIFESTYLE TOOLKIT

It is extremely important for you to be aware of your own menopause biology. If you understand your own body before menopause symptoms emerge, you can maintain your well-being balance proactively and be ahead of the game. Equally, if you understand what is happening to your body during menopause you will be better able to handle the symptoms, and your stress response will not be activated as much by the new symptoms. Knowledge and understanding will allow you to objectively identify and implement actions to alleviate symptoms.

There are many important actions that you can take to improve well-being in menopause. The disconnect is the bridge between understanding what is needed and sustainably implementing the changes required: 'I know I need to be less stressed but I don't know how I can achieve this'; 'I know I need better sleep but I cannot sleep'; 'I want to lose weight but no matter what I do my waistline is not listening.' I decided to write this book because I wanted to share my knowledge about solutions and I will provide tips, advice and strategies throughout to bridge this gap for you. All women deserve access to the knowledge required to achieve modern-day menopause health solutions.

Genes versus environment

Our genes come from our ancestors and control our instincts. Our ancestors survived famine and feast and fight and flight situations. They were hunter-gatherers and were physically active for up to 16 hours per day. Today, we are hardwired to act on their terms. We can instinctively yoyo between wanting to make large, dramatic gains and see results quickly, and resting to conserve our energy. For our ancestors this behaviour helped with survival. Endurance helped them survive war and battles, but they were much more physically active in between conflicts. Today many of us are inactive most of the time. So if we suddenly do a lot of exercise we can get injured and be put off. We can also stop at any time as exercise is barely 'needed' for daily living these days.

Our modern world has undergone a fundamental change and our genes have not had time to adjust to this shift. Even a few decades ago life was very different: there was no Internet; no overstimulating, melatonin-suppressing blue light from screens, tempting us to stay up until the small hours and disrupting sleep; there was less chronic stress as everything and everyone was less 'connected'. Only 100 years ago, our ancestors lived much shorter lives than we do now, so health risks linked to ageing, such as osteoporosis, were not historically a major issue. Bone health is now a much greater concern because we are living decades longer than even a generation ago and bones naturally grow thinner with age. Due to mass farming and soil depletion the quantity of micronutrients (vitamins and minerals), even in unprocessed food, can be poor, increasing the risk of deficiencies that can impact on health.

Well-being and quality-of-life issues in the decades after menopause were not perceived as relevant in the past, but these are crucial now. Understanding the new complex environment in our modern world can help you to understand why quick fixes and linear approaches do not tend to be sustainably effective. It also helps you to use multiple dovetailed and often simple strategies to beat your instincts and maintain or regain optimum health.

So, you see, many of your instinctive responses and coping strategies, which have long been driven by your genes, are not fit for purpose if you are to thrive in today's modern world. Embracing this concept allows you to see the world differently. For example, you would see processed food as a health threat and understand that hunger is rarely a useful protective mechanism, since more often than not you will have sufficient fat stores in the energy bank already. You would see walking and activity as protective to your muscles and bones. You would see the negative impact that technology has on your stress response and your sleep quality. When you start to understand and accept these modern-day threats, you will be able to begin to address them.

There is no quick fix

Let's go back to you, trying to make a change in your own health and well-being. You want to lose weight so you go on a diet. It's quite an extreme restriction and difficult to sustain. You are going through menopause, and the calorie restriction puts your metabolism into starvation mode. This is when your body senses that there are not enough calories coming in, so it tries to conserve energy by blocking the burning of fat. This will shut down your metabolism as your body tries to conserve energy. The end result is paradoxical – you eat less but you don't lose weight. Or at least you lose much less weight than you think you should have lost.

This is likely to be demoralising and frustrating. As you have lost weight with such a tough restriction, you think there is little point in carrying on and you go back to your old habits. Similarly, you are in menopause and decide to do a boot-camp, high-intensity training programme or the like. You get two sessions in and then sustain an injury. End of programme. You are now inactive, burning fewer calories and back to square one.

At face value these quick-fix solutions seem to be brilliant: get all the weight off in six weeks, the same weight that has gone on over several years; get fit in six weeks, having done minimal activity for ten years. It sounds like a no-brainer. Actually, it rarely, if ever, works in menopause so there is no point!

FINDING THE RIGHT BALANCE

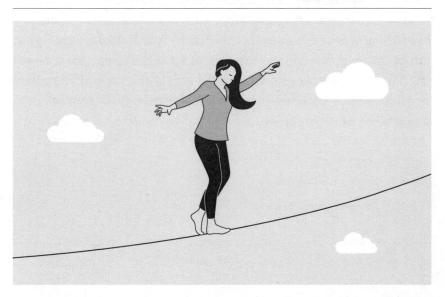

The reality about getting fit, improving sleep, lowering stress and losing weight during menopause is that for them to be sustainable, they have to be achieved through persistent, lifestyle strategies. This way, the weight does not just drop off. You will not get a flat stomach in six weeks and, to be honest, this should not be your focus. These more modest, sustainable, multifaceted lifestyle approaches take time, but will result in noticeably improved well-being before your ultimate goals are achieved.

Finding the balance can be challenging, a bit like walking a tightrope – if you lean too much one way or the other way there is a danger you will crash out – but once mastered with daily practice it can become easy. If you understand the modest changes needed to achieve your well-being goals and successfully implement them, the results will be life-changing for the long haul, and more effective than any quick fix.

A quick recap

When you start to understand the symptom trigger factors relevant to you, you will be better able to address them methodically and be your own successful menopause expert. Start tweaking your lifestyle as soon as possible, preferably ahead of perimenopause, and you will be ahead of the game. It will then be likely that symptoms will be easier to manage as your hormones start to act up. The solutions are effectively a lifestyle toolkit, detailed in Part 2. Success with these will not only make you feel better but also reduce the risk of many diseases linked to modern lifestyles.

Your Lifestyle Toolkit

CHAPTER 4

Keep Moving

I MAGINE A NEW prescription treatment with evidence showing that it improves well-being, helps with weight management, lifts mood, reduces chronic stress, strengthens muscles, improves bone strength, counteracts muscle and joint pain and injury, and regulates blood pressure and cholesterol. It also reduces the risk of heart disease, stroke, type 2 diabetes, dementia and cancer by up to 50 per cent and lowers the risk of early death by up to 30 per cent. It would be a big hit, wouldn't it? Physical activity is that prescription and it does what it says on the tin, with no downside! Building up physical activity is a positive lifestyle biohack at any time of life.

You are not built for a sedentary life – you are meant to move – but your current environment enables you to approach activity and exercise erratically. As a twenty-first-century woman going through menopause, you find yourself at probably the most challenging time of your life. This situation is unprecedented in the history of humans! You have very little time to dedicate to self-care and the first thing that tends to be dropped from the routine, when time is short, is exercise and fitness.

You can tell yourself that, because you are on the go all the time, this is a reasonable substitute for planned exercise and activity, but it is not. When you are pushing yourself with work and family commitments it is easy to neglect your own body's needs. It can be a false economy if you push yourself so much, with no time out, that you become exhausted or ill. You are likely to be more productive in work and better able to support your family if you look after yourself and keep yourself well. That is not being selfish, it's being pragmatic.

In a world in which there is a major focus on looks and appearance it is important to remember that you need to keep your insides healthy too. Physical activity can help you to achieve this. Training your mindset to find the motivation to do more activity, rather than thinking that you don't have time, is a necessary skill. Maintaining and even building up physical activity after menopause is a powerful tool to keep many modern diseases at bay, keep weight healthy, keep your stress response fit for purpose and supercharge your well-being. Exercise in menopause could be described as a panacea. It is certainly an essential element in your toolkit of holistic menopause management, to ensure ongoing well-being and vitality in the postmenopause years. This will enable you to thrive, not just survive.

MENOPAUSE NOW

As little as 50 years ago the whole Western world was more active, but things have changed. Walking levels have fallen by more than a third in the last three decades and the average person walks less than half a mile a day. The technological revolution has made cooking, cleaning, even changing the TV channel, effortless. Daily functional activity has been rendered almost obsolete. Many of us sit in a chair for most of the day, whether at home or at work, and when we travel we rarely walk to our destination.

In order to keep active these days you need to replace the functional activity that kept previous generations moving with activity that you can enjoy and sustain in the long term. It may not seem like it, but as a modern woman you are, in a way, in a favourable position with respect to activity. You can keep active in a way that suits you rather than keeping active by having to do endless chores. However, you have to remember to prioritise the time to do this.

Although your menopause experience is likely to be more challenging in many ways than your mother's and grandmothers' generation, you can enrich your well-being if you choose to, by ring-fencing time for the right type and amount of exercise for you.

A mindset to exercise

It is easy to fall short on physical activity in today's world, but that's not truly about time limitation, which many of us tell ourselves – it is about our mindset. You can use simple mind hacks to challenge your mindset and replace unhelpful thoughts with useful, motivating ones. Prioritising what's important is easier when you are mindful about it. For example, you can change the thought, 'I don't have time to exercise' to 'I can cut back five minutes of screen time here and there every day and walk instead.' Similarly, you can change the thought, 'I've heard exercise is good for health, but I forget to do it and it doesn't seem to make much difference' to 'The benefits of exercise seem invisible at first – a bit like treatment for high blood pressure – but the impact is huge and irrefutable in the long term so I will build up to do some short walks a few times a day gradually, like a lifestyle prescription.' (See Chapter 10 for more tips on mindfulness and changing your mindset.)

Pump the endorphins

You might remember a time when you, or someone you know, started a new relationship, was incredibly happy and almost effortlessly lost a significant amount of weight. This is because happy hormones trump stress hormones. Stress hormones block fat-burning and cling on to weight; endorphins have very different effects.

Endorphins are chemicals produced naturally by the nervous system. They are often called 'feel-good' hormones because they can act as pain relievers and happiness boosters. These are released when our bodies feel safe. They often peak after a successful exercise session. They are the antithesis of stress hormones! We cannot bottle them but the next best thing is adopting an exercise programme that allows their release as often as possible.

Endorphins also interact with the receptors in your brain that reduce your perception of pain. It is likely that people suffering chronic pain may have an imbalance of endorphin production.

If you can address stress and burn more calories through regular, moderate exercise or achieve a general overall increase in activity, it is likely that you will release more endorphins, experience less pain and burn more calories. And you will be well on your way to improving your well-being and health.

When overcommitment takes hold

Having taken detailed histories from thousands of women suffering from various menopausal symptoms, who I have seen in my clinics over the years, I have observed a striking common feature. I have seen strong women with unrelenting standards who are overstretched in many aspects of their lives. They push themselves very hard to do everything they feel they need to do, which can be boundless. As their hormones start changing in the context of menopause, women can sometimes struggle to achieve their demanding self-driven goals. It is conceivable that women going through the life pressures and hormone changes as they enter menopause are experiencing a type of 'overtraining syndrome'.

Overtraining syndrome encompasses a set of symptoms observed in athletes who train beyond the body's ability to recover. Athletes often exercise longer and harder so they can improve, but without adequate rest and recovery, these training regimens can backfire and actually damage performance. Conditioning requires a balance between overload and recovery. Too much overload and/

or too little recovery may result in both physical and psychological symptoms, including:

- feeling washed out, tired or drained
- general muscle and joint aches, which can be severe
- paradoxical reduced exercise tolerance
- insomnia
- headaches
- decreased immunity with more frequent infections
- irritability
- low mood
- loss of motivation
- changes in appetite
- increased susceptibility to injury

There is no research that I am aware of that demonstrates a link between overtraining and menopause. However, you probably will have noticed something very relevant about the above list – many of the symptoms described there are common symptoms in menopause. It is important to point out here that overtraining syndrome can be overcome. In almost all situations building up activity and exercise correctly can improve productivity and boost your energy and well-being immeasurably.

My Exercise Story

I was fit as a young woman, but when I started my family I felt I didn't have time for exercise. I was always busy looking after the kids and working. Exercise didn't make my shortlist of priorities and I had gradually become quite inactive. Then, when my youngest was just starting school, I developed a back problem. I started noticing pain more and more until I needed to lie down when I got home from work because the pain was so bad. I had an MRI scan of my spine and was told there was some wear and tear in my spine, and I should try using gabapentin or pregabalin for pain. Well, that was an unthinkable option for me; having observed in patients that they never support recovery, they just numb symptoms and have terrible side effects as well as being addictive, there was no way I was going to take any such drugs. I don't recommend them for my patients so I would certainly not take them myself.

Instead, I started seeing a physiotherapist. The exercises didn't make much difference to my symptoms at first but I knew it was the right approach. I then had some acupuncture, which I found amazing; I had some good relief of symptoms. Then I started doing Iyengar yoga with a wonderful teacher and, after about 18 months, my pain had gone. I realised that the modest time I spent doing the exercises was benefitting my family because it was helping me feel better and that made them happier. Not having pain made me more productive. I then built up my activity more and more. That was more than a decade ago. Nowadays I just do as much activity as I can. It energises me, boosts my mood, stops me having any pain, de-stresses me and helps my brain focus. I cannot recommend any lifestyle approach more highly than exercise.

TOP TIP: BENEFITS OF REGULAR PHYSICAL ACTIVITY

- Reduces your risk of a heart attack.
- Manages your weight better.
- Lowers blood cholesterol level.
- Lowers the risk of type 2 diabetes and some cancers.
- Lowers blood pressure.
- Strengthens bones, muscles and joints, and lowers the risk of developing osteoporosis.
- Lowers your risk of falling.

STARTING A NEW EXERCISE ROUTINE

The best way to achieve the right approach to activity in menopause is to embark upon a gradual build-up of physical activity, consolidate it and then maintain it. How much activity that will be, and how long the build-up process will take, will depend on your current fitness level. You must feel comfortable with the approach you are taking. If it feels too difficult, or if you get injured, that means it is too much too fast. Reflecting on how well your exercise programme is going is very important. Maintaining an injury-free system is the target and modifying your activity programme to ensure you stay injury free is key.

Take small steps

As menopause progresses, it is more important than ever to maintain a good level of fitness in order to stay active, healthy and independent throughout the rest of your life. Nearly every woman knows that exercise is good. However, it is often difficult to convert that knowledge into action. Self-doubt can creep in – 'Everyone is fitter than me', 'It will be too hard', 'I'm so unfit that I don't know where to start!' The thing to remember is that we all start somewhere, and anything will be better than nothing. Even for regular exercisers, stepping out of the door can be the hardest thing. But small steps can make sustainable gains; make a short-term plan – what you will do and when – and stick to it. Then keep making those small plans and sticking to them. Don't think too much of the bigger picture, just the small, hugely positive steps that you are taking each time you step out of the door and do more exercise than you have done before. Be positive and kind to yourself, recognising the small goals that you achieve. This approach will help you to reach your longer-term goal, rather than being defeated by the enormity of it.

Take some time to reflect on what you are doing currently. For example, if you walk the dog for 30 minutes per day, you could start with a light programme of exercise, once or twice a week, of a similar length. Next, do something you enjoy. If you have hated swimming all your life, you are unlikely to stick at it. There are lots of different things to try these days (see page 47 for some ideas). Many of us admit to spending significant amounts of time looking at screens for leisure, admin or work purposes. Try to siphon off a fraction of this time and dedicate it to 'micro' exercise opportunities. Twenty extra minutes a day moving would make a positive long-term difference.

When Sir Dave Brailsford became performance director of British Cycling, he set about breaking down the objective of winning races into its component parts, utilising the concept of 'marginal gains'. The marginal gains theory is concerned with small incremental improvements in any process, which, when added together, make a significant improvement. This ingenious approach to sporting success is a perfect allegory for long-term menopause strength and fitness. Essentially, small gradual changes in activity and movement result in a significant and sustainable incremental improvement.

Set realistic goals

Being objective is important when trying to build up activity. Setting personal goals and regularly re-evaluating them is very helpful. Goals should be 'SMART': specific, measurable, achievable, rewarding and time limited. The table below shows how your goal-setting can influence whether you will persevere with the activity:

SMART goals

Goal	Expectation	Likely to succeed	Likely to quit
Specific	Is your goal clear or too vague?	I will set a realistic daily walking time, stick to it and build by small increments each week	I am going to get fit

Goal	Expectation	Likely to succeed	Likely to quit
Measurable	How will you know if you have achieved your goal?	I will use a wearable smart watch, make a spreadsheet or use a fitness app to track my steps and active time	I will go for a run when I have time
Achievable	How likely are you to be successful?	I want to build up to X minutes' walking every day	I have not done any exercise for a while but I am going to sign up for a 10-k run
Rewarding	Will you enjoy the results?	I love walking outdoors	I have never done running regularly in my life
Time limited	When do you want to have achieved your goal?	I will aim for building up over 6 weeks	The 10-k run is in 4 weeks

The most important advice is to do activities that you enjoy because then you will be more likely to stick at them.

There are many options to keep you active in menopause, including walking, swimming, cycling, dancing, aerobics, weightlifting, pump classes ... the list goes on. If you have done a particular activity or sport a lot before that you have enjoyed, your muscles and joints may take to that more easily than something you have never done. Enjoyment is key; that is the reward with exercise and we must ensure lots of enjoyment through menopause.

Toning and strengthening exercises are particularly important because they strengthen all the muscles. These include squats, lunges and arm-raise exercises with small weights, repeated in sets, and are really useful functional exercises. There are many ways to tone and strengthen. These and activities like yoga and Pilates are functional training approaches. Functional training tends to strengthen all the muscle groups, which can weaken if you spend a lot of time sitting down, and can help make everyday activities like bending down, getting up off the floor and general housework feel easier to do.

Cardio exercise, such as cycling, running and dancing, is great for the heart and blood vessels but can result in muscle and joint injuries if the exercise is attempted for the first time during menopause and is built up too quickly. These activities should also be very cautiously approached in people with known heart problems and high blood pressure.

Swimming is both toning and cardiovascular. It is therefore a really good option for people who like being in the water. If you don't like swimming, it is probably not a suitable exercise to start in menopause, as it is human nature to tend to persevere with activities you enjoy and quit those you don't. And whatever activity you choose, the aim is not to quit!

Walking is a very underrated physical activity with fantastic health benefits. It is the one activity that most people of any age can participate in. It offers various levels of challenge depending on the fitness level of the individual. It is clear from evidence that even people with painful hip and knee arthritis benefit from walking. Outcomes are improved for people with many health problems who choose to remain active and build up activity. With leg and foot pain issues, walking for short periods is often tolerated well and short walks can be repeated several times per day with rests in between to allow a reasonable daily total number of steps. The current health guide is to aim for 10,000 steps per day, which, although challenging, can be achieved, even as you get older, with the right positive mindset. Slow and steady *can* win the race.

In the following table I have listed several different levels of baseline activity so you can identify which one describes you best. I have then set an initial goal (Do's) and then something you can work up to gradually, using your SMART goals (Do more). The 'Don't' column shows some dangers and pitfalls that you should be wary of. If you complete one level successfully you can move to the next level up.

How to build up exercise and activity in menopause

Level	Do's	Do more	Don't
Couch potato	Try a 5–10-minute brisk walk, to get your breathing and heart rate up. Do it 3–4 times a day if you can, every day	Slowly build up to 30 minutes' brisk walking every day	Don't try to do too much if your starting point in menopause is zero. Couch to 5k may be too much
Pottering all the time but no regular activity	Plan regular activity, such as a regular walk or a gentle gym programme	Build up gradually. Avoid overdoing it, getting injured and ending up back at square one	Don't procrastinate because you are too busy. We are all busy!

Level	Do's	Do more	Don't
Walking the dog	Track walking times. If you do more than 10,000 steps per day you are doing well. You could add in some gentle core exercise	Keep it regular, and you can build up if time allows	Don't stop
Gym 1–3 times per week	Continue and do some walking in between gym sessions – aim for 10,000 steps per day	Build up the intensity of exercise gradually	Don't get injured; be cautious with any new programme or class
Gym bunny (4 or more times per week)	Continue and walk in between exercise sessions. Try to keep above 10,000 steps per day	Not necessary if you are going to the gym more than 3 times per week and walking 10,000 steps per day	Don't get injured; be cautious with any new programme or class
Long-distance running/high-level training/triathlons	Try to maintain this level	Maintaining is the key	Don't stop; be cautious about injury

The power of the pelvic floor

Adult women of any age can develop pelvic floor problems and these can be common after pregnancy. Pelvic floor exercises and strengthening benefit bladder and bowel function and reduce risk of prolapse. They can reduce leakage, incontinence, urgency and the risk of urinary tract infections (UTIs). They can also reduce vaginal and pelvic pain during sex and improve the sexual experience. Yoga and Pilates are brilliant at strengthening your core muscles and your pelvic floor.

Here is how to do a Kegel pelvic floor exercise:

1. With an empty bladder, tighten your bladder and bowel muscles as if you are trying to stop yourself passing urine or wind.
2. Hold tight and count 3–5 seconds.
3. Relax the muscles and count 3–5 seconds.
4. Repeat up to 10 times, up to 3 times a day. Even if you repeat a fraction of that number it's better than nothing!

Preventing Injury

If you have never had an injury by the time of menopause you are truly lucky! Injury is a very common pitfall encountered in all physical training programmes at any age and for males and females alike. In menopause, muscles and joints will generally be stiffer and take longer to warm up. It is therefore very important to warm up gently before exercise. This simple step can help prevent muscle injuries. Gentle yoga and Pilates are particularly good because they have a low risk of injury when starting from scratch. They can be successfully practised at any age and give you a total body workout.

If you are generally inactive, it is easy to inadvertently overdo activity when you first make lifestyle changes. If, for example, you spend most of your time with your arms in front of you typing on a computer, then you suddenly decide to have a game of tennis for the first time in years, which involves lifting your arms and shoulders and forcefully pounding a ball with the racket, you could easily sustain a shoulder injury. Once injured you may be out of action for a while, which is exactly what you must try to avoid.

High-intensity programmes are popular personal training approaches, because in many circumstances this approach leads to rapid progress with fitness. However, women in menopause need to be wary of these approaches because the muscles and joints in menopause are not set up for a rapid building up of fitness. Slow and steady is much safer and better for you. Be warned that intensive fitness programmes that you are not used to could induce an injury that ducks you out of exercise for months.

Regular functional activity approaches, maintaining a good daily level of movement and not overdoing it (avoiding overtraining) is the winning approach. Choosing the right activity and the right level and building up gradually is key. It is human nature to push yourself; holding back is not instinctive and it can be very hard to do. You need to be mindful that less can be more with the right approach and it is possible to be stronger and less injury-prone after menopause than before it.

If you are forewarned about the risks of injury with the right information you will be more likely to be cautious with any new exercise programme and protect your joints and muscles, limiting the risk of damage. Avoiding injury is not the same as avoiding activity. It is about managing activity and making changes gradually.

If you do get an injury it is important to keep perspective. You had the right idea but the delivery was not on-target. Injuries and pain can be demoralising and can sometimes aggravate other menopause symptoms. If you have an injury you should consider seeking professional advice. Physiotherapy is very important in recovering from an injury. Trying to keep movement going for all the other muscles and joints while the injury recovers is crucial at any time of life including menopause This will prevent all the other muscles from weakening while you are out of action (known as disuse atrophy), which at worst can result in a vicious cycle of weakness and reduced function, and could make it harder to build up once the injury recovers.

It is important to remember that everyone's biology and environment are different. If you are at the height of your fitness going

DISUSE ATROPHY

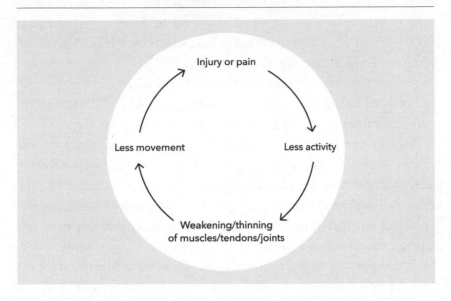

through menopause, you may not notice any change in performance; after all, you have learned all the tools to prevent injury along the way and you can simply carry on seamlessly through menopause.

On the other hand, if you have been very inactive all your adult life, perhaps spending hours each day sitting in a busy desk job, you will need to be careful about building up activity if you are starting this in menopause. You may be more likely to get menopause aches and pains, which could instinctively put you off doing activity. I caution against this. Less activity begets less activity and this is unlikely to result in any positive long-term gain in menopause.

A quick recap

The secret of getting activity management right in menopause is different for everyone and will be governed by your premenopausal fitness level, your overall approach to physical activity and whether you encounter any setbacks.

Very gradual incremental activity, following the principle of marginal gains theory, is safe, effective and unlikely to cause injury. This will allow gradual build-up of fitness and stamina. High-intensity activity and rapid training programmes are more likely to induce injuries and set back well-being in menopause. If the only exercise you can do is walking, be reassured that the majority of health and well-being benefits associated with exercise can be achieved by walking at least 30 minutes every day.

Increasing activity is a precise science (at any time in life) but once learned can be easy. If you have been sedentary all your adult life, and then conquer the skill of regular physical activity without injury as you enter menopause, you are likely to feel better and be healthier in many respects during menopause than you have felt through your whole adult life.

It's important to bear in mind that fitness is a lifestyle with no finish line. If you are mindful about this throughout life, and get your activity programme right, you will seamlessly maintain your fitness level during menopause and be less susceptible to injury going forward. Your sense of balance will be better and your bones will be stronger. Decades later you will remain stronger and be much less susceptible to falls and broken bones.

CHAPTER 5

An A to Z of Nutrients in Menopause

NUTRITION IS EXCEPTIONALLY important during menopause. To keep healthy, feel well, avoid weight gain and reduce your risk of long-term health problems, what you eat matters. If you eat predominantly natural, unprocessed foods from a variety of different food groups, you will already be well on your way to obtaining the nutrients you need. With a diet rich in healthy food your portion sizes can generally be larger than with more processed meals. Natural, unprocessed food keeps you feeling fuller for longer, prevents sugar and energy crashes, reduces fluid retention and bloating, and protects against many preventable diseases. Achieving nutritional balance in menopause can also help with your energy, well-being, bone health, skin, hair and nail quality.

In this chapter I want to inform you about the health benefits that some important essential nutrients provide for menopause health. I will explain the health impact of nutrient deficiencies and how you can identify and address them. You also need to be aware that you can sometimes get too much of a good thing! But first let's be clear on what nutrients are and why they are important.

Nutrients are compounds in foods that are essential to life and health, providing you with energy, the building blocks for cell repair and function, and the substances necessary to regulate chemical processes. The major nutrient groups are carbohydrates, fat and protein (collectively known as 'macronutrients'), vitamins and minerals (collectively known as 'micronutrients'), and water. You need the right amount of all of these for your body to function properly and stay healthy. Having too much or not enough can cause health problems so good nutrition is a fine balance.

There is a summary of the types of food that you should try to include in your diet on a daily basis and what may be consumed less frequently in Appendix 1 (page 245). To give you some general ideas and inspiration, Appendix 2 (page 248) shows a sample menu that gives examples of meals that contain a wide variety of nutrients that are beneficial for menopause health.

MACRONUTRIENTS: FAT, CARBOHYDRATES AND PROTEIN

Fat

Fat tends to have a reputation for being bad for your health, but it is the *type* of fat that matters. Your body needs some fat because it helps you absorb some vitamins and minerals. It is also important for blood clotting, muscle movement and inflammation, as well as being a major source of energy.

A balanced diet should include monounsaturated and polyunsaturated fats, which can be found in plant sources of fat, such as avocados, olive oil, nuts and seeds, as well as oily fish. They contain essential fatty acids and are really good for you.

Fatty acids

Omega-3 fatty acids are essential fats. They have important benefits for your heart, brain and metabolism. They are anti-inflammatory and have a role in heart health, brain function and mood. They are found in fish and fish oil, flaxseed, chia seeds, walnuts, edamame and kidney beans, and tofu.

Omega-6 fatty acids are essential fats that are an important source of energy. These are found in vegetable oils, nuts and seeds. Western diets tend to contain too many of these. They promote inflammation. A diet that includes balanced amounts of omega-3 and -6 fatty acids may reduce inflammation.

Omega-9 fatty acids are non-essential fats, as they can be produced by the body. They have been shown to increase good cholesterol and decrease bad cholesterol. They are found in nuts and vegetable oils.

Saturated fat

Saturated fat is obtained from meat and dairy products and also trans fats, which are synthetic fats used to make some processed foods. Eating too much of these types of fat can cause high cholesterol, weight gain, heart and blood vessel disease, and cancer.

Carbs

There are different types of carbs and the difference mainly relates to how quickly they can release sugar from your gut into your blood.

Rapid-release carbs include processed starchy food, stripped of their fibre, including white bread, pasta and pastry, and all sugars, such as sweets, chocolate, biscuits, cakes and sugary drinks. They release energy quickly and can spike your blood sugar. While this may be helpful if you are burning a lot of calories, for example during intensive exercise, in most situations in our modern world our sugar and starch consumption is excessive. It can tend to give you a short-term energy boost, so can feel gratifying to your appetite centre, but then causes a sugar crash later, making you want to eat more of the same.

Slow-release carbs have a very different effect. Starchy foods that are less processed and contain more natural fibre, such as wholegrain options, are slower to absorb into your bloodstream and provide a more sustained release of energy. They do not spike your blood sugar and they keep your appetite in check for longer. They can keep hunger at bay and reduce energy crashes as your blood sugar falls. They appear to be good for your heart, blood vessels and cholesterol, and keep brain function and focus sharp. The best of the slow-release carbs, and at the opposite end of rapid-release carbs, is dietary fibre. This has major health benefits and is plentiful in unprocessed foods.

Modern diets containing a lot of processed food are low in dietary fibre. Processed food is being consumed in epidemic quantities today, and you may not always be aware that you are consuming it.

TOP TIP: THE PROBLEM WITH PROCESSED FOODS

Some, but not all, processed food may be fortified with certain nutrients, but these foods are not nutritionally balanced. If they are the main type of food you consume, they will not provide you with the nutritional balance you need for long-term health. Processed foods are constructed to be desirable to our palate and contain a greater proportion of sugar, fat, salt, preservatives and sometimes cancer-causing chemicals.

Fibre

Fibre refers to the plant-based carbs and other food sources that cannot be digested. Its importance is often under-recognised. It is crucially important in maintaining the right balance of bacteria in your gut, the so-called 'gut microbiome'. Fibre is present in all plant-based foods, including fruit, vegetables, grains, nuts, seeds and pulses. It is also found in shellfish. Fibre comes in two types: soluble and insoluble. Most plant foods contain some of each kind of fibre.

Soluble fibre slows digestion and helps you absorb nutrients from food. By slowing digestion, soluble fibre can slow the absorption of fat, sugar and starch, which can help lower blood cholesterol and blood sugar levels. These are all good effects to support a healthy menopause.

Insoluble fibre adds bulk to your stool and supports your gut health and function, so it can be of benefit to you if you struggle with constipation or irregular stools. Natural foods containing fibre also contain many essential micronutrients and these are all the more important in menopause.

High dietary fibre intake has many benefits during menopause. It protects against several preventable diseases, such as heart disease, type 2 diabetes and bowel cancer, and reduces your overall long-term health risks. High-fibre diets also help with weight loss, which is usually a welcome effect during menopause.

Women need 20–30g of dietary fibre per day. Appendix 3 (page 250) shows which foods contain fibre and how much, so you can see if you have enough on a daily basis. If not, you can increase the amount you eat by choosing foods from the fibre list that you enjoy eating and adding them in wherever possible.

A high-fibre diet usually improves symptoms of chronic constipation. However, if you have other gut or pelvic floor issues, increased dietary fibre may not produce the desired results. If this is the case, it is best to seek advice from a healthcare professional. Adjustment to an increase in fibre may take time, even when you have no major gut problem, and your gut may struggle with the change initially. It is therefore wise to make the change gradually.

> ### TOP TIP: HOW TO MAKE HEALTHY TREATS
>
> When baking, you can substitute 50–100g of flour for ground almonds in most sweet baking recipes, likes cakes and muffins, to add vitamins, minerals, protein and fibre to your recipe.

Protein

Your body uses protein to build and repair tissues. You also use protein to make enzymes, hormones and other chemical messengers. Protein is an important building block of bones, muscles, cartilage, skin and blood. An adequate intake of protein is important to maintain your muscle and bone strength through menopause. Protein is an appetite suppressant, so not eating enough could mean that you crave carbs. The recommended daily amount of protein is approximately 45–50g per day, which is about two palm-sized portions of meat, fish, tofu, nuts or pulses. Appendix 3 (page 250) lists some common foods that contain protein so you can see if you are eating enough protein each day. If you are not, you should try to increase it by adding in some of the foods listed.

MICRONUTRIENTS: VITAMINS AND MINERALS

A micronutrient is an element or substance required in trace amounts for the normal and healthy functioning of all the systems in your body. These cannot be made in adequate amounts in your body so need to be obtained from food sources. Examples that may be familiar to you are vitamins and minerals. Essential micronutrients are building blocks for energy, well-being and overall health.

MENOPAUSE NOW

In an ideal world, the best way to get vitamins and minerals is from a well-rounded diet, with plenty of fruits, vegetables, pulses, whole grains and lean sources of protein, along with healthy fat sources, such as nuts and olive oil. The problem is that we don't live in an ideal world and few of us have a perfect approach to nutrition. That can link with our instincts craving sugar and fat. But also in the mix is mass farming and soil depletion, which have come with globalisation. This means that mass-produced natural foods may not contain the micronutrient content that is expected. Crops grown decades ago were richer in vitamins and minerals than the varieties most of us consume today.

Severe vitamin and mineral deficiencies are considered to be rare today in the modern world. However, eating less than optimal amounts of foods containing important vitamins, minerals and other nutrients has been linked to a number of major illnesses, such as heart disease, type 2 diabetes, cancer, dementia and osteoporosis. These are really important risks to consider in menopause and are relatively easy to address.

There are 13 essential vitamins and 15 or more essential minerals (often described as 'A to Zinc'). Each one has an essential role, and having the right amount of these in your body is very important for a healthy menopause. They are needed all the more in menopause to keep all the body systems functioning well. This is partly because there are increased requirements during menopause, but also possibly because of reduced absorption from the gut. Other health issues and use of medicines can sometimes interfere with vitamin and mineral absorption and metabolism. It is not uncommon to have insufficient amounts in your diet, and alcohol reduces absorption of several vitamins and minerals. Several diseases can be caused or worsened by vitamin and mineral deficiencies.

The 13 essential vitamins are: vitamins A, C, D, E, K and the B vitamins: thiamine (B1), riboflavin (B2), niacin (B3), pantothenic acid (B5), pyroxidine (B6), biotin (B7), folate (B9) and cobalamin (B12).

The water-soluble vitamins (all the B vitamins and vitamin C) are easily absorbed into the body but are not stored, so need to be consumed regularly to maintain good levels as they are removed from the body in your urine. The exception to this is vitamin B12, which is the only water-soluble vitamin that can be stored in the liver.

Fat-soluble vitamins can be stored in the liver and in fatty tissues and released from stores gradually. The fat-soluble vitamins include A, D, E and K.

Of the essential minerals, some are needed in relatively large amounts, such as calcium, sodium, potassium, phosphorus, magnesium and chloride, while others are only needed in trace amounts – the so-called 'trace elements'. The essential minerals have a wide range of important functions to keep your menopause healthy.

Below is a guide to why you need fibre, protein and each essential vitamin and mineral, and the best food sources from which to obtain them. Each has an essential role in menopause for hormone health, well-being and to protect against several diseases. You may find it difficult to remember all the vitamin and minerals, what they are found in and what they do, so if you look at the 'To inspire you' column you can identify which health benefits you are specifically interested in and work back to increase those nutrients in your diet.

Nutrient essentials: Foods that support health and well-being in menopause

Nutrient	Found in	To inspire you
Fibre: aim for 20–30g per day – a mixture of soluble and insoluble fibre		
Soluble fibre	Apples, barley, beans, carrots, citrus fruits, oat bran, oats, peas, potatoes, rice, strawberries (see Appendix 1)	It slows digestion and helps you absorb nutrients from food. It can help lower cholesterol and glucose levels. All fibre is associated with reduced risk of some diseases such as cardiovascular disease, type 2 diabetes and bowel cancer. A crucial nutrient in menopause
Insoluble fibre	Beans, such as green beans, nuts, potato skin and the skins of many fruits and vegetables, vegetables, such as cauliflower, wheat bran, wholegrain cereals, wholewheat flour (see Appendix 1)	Adds bulk to your stool, so helps with constipation. Reduces risk of bowel cancer and helps manage diverticular disease
Protein: aim for 45–50g per day	Eggs, fish, meat, nuts, oats, pulses, seeds, tofu (see Appendix 2)	Helps with your muscle and bone strength, reduces your appetite and cravings

Nutrient	Found in	To inspire you
Vitamin A (retinol)	Egg yolks, fortified dairy products, salmon and other cold-water fish. Carrots contain beta-carotene, which is a precursor of vitamin A	Promotes healthy skin, hair, nails, gums, glands, bones and teeth. It is important for vision. It may help prevent lung cancer
Vitamin B1 (thiamine)	Beef, brown rice, eggs, legumes*, liver, milk, nuts, oats, oranges, peas, pork, seeds, soymilk, watermelons, yeast	Needed for healthy skin, hair, muscles and brain, and is critical for nerve function
Vitamin B2 (riboflavin)	Dairy products, fortified cereals and grains, fortified soy/rice, green vegetables, lean meat, poultry, raw mushrooms	Aids adrenal function, supports normal vision and helps maintain healthy skin
Vitamin B3 (niacin)	Fish, fortified and whole grains, meat, mushrooms, peanut butter, potatoes, poultry	Essential for healthy skin, blood cells, brain and nervous system. In large doses, vitamin B3 can lower cholesterol
Vitamin B5 (pantothenic acid)	Avocados, broccoli, cereals, eggs, fortified breads, lean meats, milk, mushrooms, poultry, seafood, tomatoes, whole grains	This helps make fats, neurotransmitters, steroid hormones and haemoglobin. It aids energy metabolism and normal blood sugar levels

Nutrient	Found in	To inspire you
Vitamin B6 (pyridoxine)	Bananas, cereals, fish, grains, green leafy vegetables, meat, potatoes, poultry, soybeans	May lower the risk of heart disease. It assists in fatty acids and protein metabolism. It supports normal growth of nerve cells. It has a role in making red blood cells and DNA
Vitamin B7 (biotin)	Egg yolks, fish, nuts, soybeans, whole grains, yeast	Needed for healthy bones and strong, healthy hair
Vitamin B9 (folic acid)	Asparagus, avocados, black-eyed peas, chickpeas, fortified flour, fortified grains and cereals, leafy green vegetables, liver, okra, orange juice, tomato juice, yeast	Supports the manufacture of DNA, RNA, red blood cells and certain amino acids
Vitamin B12 (cobalamin)	Cheese, eggs, fish, fortified cereals, fortified soymilk, meat, milk, poultry	May lower the risk of heart disease. It protects nerve cells and encourages their normal growth. It helps make red blood cells and DNA
Vitamin C (ascorbic acid)	Bell peppers, broccoli, Brussels sprouts, citrus fruits, fruit juices (especially citrus), potatoes, spinach, strawberries, tomatoes	May lower the risk for some cancers. May protect against cataracts. Helps make collagen. Helps make serotonin and noradrenaline. Acts as an antioxidant. Supports immune function

Nutrient	Found in	To inspire you
Vitamin D (calciferol)	Sunlight (made in the skin when exposed to the sun); also fortified cereals and dairy products, oily fish	Essential for healthy teeth and bones. It is a hormone and has important immune system beneficial effects
Vitamin E	Eggs, fortified cereals, leafy green vegetables, margarine, nuts, seeds, vegetable oils, wheat germ, whole grains	An antioxidant, may protect against Alzheimer's disease
Vitamin K	Broccoli, eggs, kale and other green leafy vegetables, liver, milk, spinach, sprouts	Plays a role in blood clotting, bone metabolism and regulating blood calcium levels
Calcium	Cheese, fortified juices, leafy green vegetables, such as broccoli and kale, milk, salmon, sardines, tofu, yoghurt	Builds and protects bones and teeth. It supports muscle function
Chloride	Processed foods, salt (sodium chloride), soy sauce	Balances fluids in the body
Chromium	Cheese, eggs, fish, meat, nuts, potatoes, poultry, some cereals	Helps maintain normal blood glucose levels and is needed to free energy from glucose

Nutrient	Found in	To inspire you
Copper	Beans, black pepper, cocoa, liver, nuts, prunes, seeds, shellfish, wholegrain products	Maintains healthy bones, blood vessels, nerves and immune function. Contributes to iron absorption
Fluoride	Marine fish, toothpaste with fluoride, water that is fluoridated	Protects against dental cavities
Iodine	Iodised salt, seafood	Essential for a healthy thyroid gland to balance the body's metabolism
Iron	Eggs, fortified bread and grain products, fruits, green vegetables, poultry, red meat	Essential for transporting oxygen throughout the body
Magnesium	Cashews, green vegetables, such as spinach and broccoli, legumes*, halibut, milk, sunflower seeds and other seeds, wholewheat bread	Helps maintain normal nerve and muscle function, supports a healthy immune system, keeps the heartbeat steady and helps bones and teeth remain strong
Manganese	Fish, legumes*, nuts, tea, whole grains	Important for bone formation and metabolism
Molybdenum	Grain products, legumes*, milk, nuts	Removes toxins from the body

Nutrient	Found in	To inspire you
Phosphorus	Almonds, broccoli, eggs, fish, green peas, liver, meat, milk and dairy products, potatoes, poultry	Supports healthy bones and teeth
Selenium	Grain products, organ meats, seafood, walnuts; sometimes other nuts (depends on soil content)	Prevents cell damage, important for healthy thyroid gland function
Sodium	Salt	Balances fluids in the body, but most people have too much
Sulphur	Protein-rich foods, such as fish, legumes*, meats, nuts, poultry	Needed for healthy hair, skin and nails
Zinc	Beans, fortified cereals, nuts, oysters and some other seafood, poultry, red meat	Essential for a healthy functioning immune system

*Examples of legumes include: beans, peas, chickpeas, lentils and peanuts.

WATER

Keeping well hydrated in menopause is essential for every cell in your body to function well. It is also important for kidney function. Dehydration can result in dizziness, which can put you at risk of falls. It is possible to drink too much water and that can make you need to use the bathroom at night and can cause your bladder to be more irritable.

It may be easier to become dehydrated as you get older and complications of dehydration can result in hospital admissions, which can set back your overall health. Prevention is better than cure. Try to ensure you drink no less than 1.2 litres and up to 3 litres of fluid per day depending on your exercise level, sweating level and weather temperature.

> **KEY FACT**
>
> Dehydration in older people is a major health risk. It can cause sunken skin, kidney problems, low blood pressure, dizziness, fatigue, confusion and falls.

SUPPLEMENTS

A common perception is that if you eat enough food then you will get all the nutrients you need and won't need to worry specifically about adding any particular types of nutritional supplements. I believe that, in many circumstances today, this is a misconception.

If you like the idea of a biohack to enhance your energy, well-being and risks of preventable diseases, optimising your micronutrient levels with a single complete A to Z general supplement to support a healthy diet appears to be a logical and helpful approach with no risk of harm, apart from the cost of the tablet. Good supplements tend to contain around 50–100 per cent of the recommended daily amount of essential vitamins and minerals – in these quantities you will not 'overdose' even if you have a good diet. There are many brands available in all high-street pharmacies. It's worth noting that the supplements specifically branded for menopause tend to be more costly and don't usually have a significant advantage over other A to Z supplements. Supplements should always be taken with a meal to be digested properly. It is, however, very important to acknowledge that a supplement is never a substitute for a balanced diet. It can only support a healthy balanced diet as a fail-safe back-up or add-on.

There are lots of other supplements that are not classed as essential but which many people seem to gain benefit from in menopause. I will discuss some of these complementary supplements and remedies in Chapter 13.

ORGANIC FOOD

The jury is still out as to whether organic food is better for you. You cannot assume that if you only eat organic food you will have enough of everything you need. Organic food will certainly contain fewer harmful chemicals. Organic meat and dairy contain about 50 per cent more omega-3 fatty acids, and studies suggest organic meat and vegetables contain greater quantities of anti-oxidants (anti-cancer substances). However, organic crops do not appear to contain higher levels of vitamins. Protein levels have also been found to be lower in some organic crops. Organic dairy produce contains 35–40 per cent less iodine than non-organic conventional dairy sources.

If you like the environmental benefits of organic agriculture, the greater proportion of antioxidants and omega-3 fatty acids and fewer chemicals will logically have some beneficial health effects.

FERMENTED FOOD

Fermented foods are said to be rich in probiotic bacteria, so by consuming these foods you are adding beneficial bacteria and enzymes to your overall gut flora, increasing the health of your gut microbiome and digestive system, and enhancing the immune system. Examples of fermented foods are: kimchi, sauerkraut, kefir, tempeh, kombucha, olives and live yoghurt. These foods may also reduce heart disease risk and aid digestion, immunity and weight loss.

PLANT-BASED EATING

The decision about what sort of diet to follow is very individual but the most important factor from a health perspective is to make sure that your nutritional intake is balanced. For health, it's important for everyone to try to include a wide variety of fruits, vegetables and whole grains in their diet.

Many people are now turning to vegetarian and vegan life-styles due to the potential health benefits as well as environmental sustainability and animal welfare. Flexible plant-based eating is recognised as not only nutritionally sufficient but also as a way to reduce the risk of many chronic illnesses. If you choose to be totally vegetarian or vegan you should be proactive in ensuring that you are able to obtain all the essential micronutrients and macronutrients from your diet, and if there is anything missing you will need to supplement appropriately.

There are some potential deficiencies that can be associated with vegetarian diets, including vitamin B12, iodine, iron and protein. These can easily be optimised or added as supplements as long as you know what's needed (see above).

In a similar way, those carnivores who love meat need to be aware of the potential negative health effects of processed meat and saturated meat fats, and if meat eaters don't eat enough vege-tables they can also become deficient in several vitamins.

Veganism differs from vegetarianism in that this approach is dairy- and egg-free, as well as being meat- and fish-free. In addition to potential extra nutrients that may be needed for vege-tarians, vegans also need to be mindful about ensuring enough calcium intake because most people get much of their calcium from dairy sources. It is easy to adopt a dairy-free diet and not compensate enough to maintain calcium intake. This can run the risk of premature bone thinning and fractures. However, these days it is easy to get enough calcium with a vegan diet because most dairy-alternative milk products are fortified with calcium. They are more expensive than cow's milk though. It is knowing about and mitigating these potential risks that matters.

Diets that are very low in calcium represent a public health issue as you get older because these can significantly increase the risk of osteoporosis. Osteoporotic hip fractures have a high complication rate in older age. We'll talk more about calcium and bone health in Chapter 12.

People choosing to be vegan, who are not aware of these crucial nutritional facts, could choose to live on processed vegan foods (vegan pizza, sweets, chips, bread and pasta) and perceive these to be healthy because they are vegan. They will get enough calories with this processed approach and if they are gaining weight they could easily mistakenly think they are getting everything they need. But this diet (without appropriate supplementation) could lead to micronutrient deficiencies and potential negative health consequences.

An increasingly popular dietary approach is a flexitarian diet, also referred to as 'casual vegetarianism'. This involves an increased intake of plant-based meals without completely eliminating meat, fish or dairy. It is about adding new natural foods to your diet as opposed to excluding any. This can be beneficial for health and doesn't seem to have a downside.

You can get many of the health benefits of being vegetarian without going all the way. This is very much following a Mediterranean eating pattern, which is known to be associated with longer life and reduced risk of several diseases. It is simply a predominantly unprocessed, plant-based diet with a sparing use of meat and fish. Even if you don't want to become a complete vegetarian, you can steer your diet in that direction with a few simple substitutions, such as plant-based sources of protein, for example beans or tofu, or fish instead of meat a couple of times a week.

A quick recap

Nutrition is very important to maintain a healthy menopause. What you eat can have an impact on well-being, gut health, weight management and many preventable and serious diseases. Mild deficiencies of essential micronutrients, dietary fibre and essential fatty acids are relatively common and you may be more at risk from these deficiencies during menopause.

If you have persistent menopause symptoms, such as fatigue, brain fog or bloating, if you are under a lot of stress or if your diet is limited, you should consider taking a daily supplement with your main meal. A standard A to Z supplement should include an adequate replacement dose of all the essential vitamins and minerals, possibly with the exception of enough vitamin D. I will talk more about vitamin D in Chapter 12 (page 162).

CHAPTER 6

Fighting Flushes and Sweats

T HE MOST NOTORIOUS symptoms of menopause are hot flushes (called 'flashes' in the US) and sweats. Flushes are experienced very individually. You may simply notice a warm sensation that moves over your whole body and which is untroublesome, or you may experience an intense warmth that quickly spreads across your whole body and face and can feel like being enclosed in a furnace. The symptom typically lasts for several minutes but can persist for longer and can be accompanied or followed by intense sweating. Sweating can also occur without the typical flush. The episodes can happen day or night and can be occasional or relentless. About 70–80 per cent of women will experience these symptoms to some extent during menopause. Most menopausal symptoms last 2–10 years, but the duration is very variable and this holds true for hot flushes and night sweats. Occasionally these can be lifelong after menopause, but for most women they gradually settle with time.

Night sweats and hot flushes are renowned for disrupting sleep. At worst, you might need to change your bedclothes several times per night because the sweats are drenching and therefore your sleep quality, and often that of your partner, can be disrupted.

Daytime episodes can trigger anxiety, palpitations, poor concentration and poor focus, and can very be embarrassing if sweat is dripping down your face, chest or back. These symptoms can be really troublesome in the workplace.

> ### MENOPAUSE NOW
>
> Women in menopause represent the fastest growing demographic in the UK workforce and the number of women over 50 years in employment has risen by 50 per cent in the last 30 years. Hot flushes are a major issue for women at work and have been linked to women having a higher intention to leave the workforce early.

TREATMENT OPTIONS

More than half of all women approaching menopause will seek treatment for troublesome hot flushes and sweats. Many will choose to try natural measures rather than turning to prescription medication initially.

There is a lot of confusion around this area and there are many non-proven treatments available, not infrequently costly, using targeted advertising, facilitated by social media. However, there are a number of practical strategies that can make a difference to the severity of symptoms. Avoiding certain triggers for hot sweats and flushes and other practical approaches can help reduce your symptoms and have no downsides, so are worth a try.

Avoiding triggers including spicy food, hot drinks and too much alcohol, stressful situations, tight, restrictive clothing, hot environments and cigarette smoke (even passive) are very helpful strategies, and steering clear of these situations can lessen the frequency of symptoms.

Keeping cool is a no-brainer because slight increases in your body's core temperature can trigger hot flushes. Having iced water or tea rather than hot coffee is a simple technique that can reduce symptoms. If you feel a hot flush coming on, sip a cold drink. Lower the room temperature, if you can – open windows or use a fan or air conditioner. Portable or desk fans can be very helpful for easing symptoms once they begin.

Wearing loose layers (avoid polo necks) so that you can rapidly de-clothe if needed during the day, sticking to lightweight, loose-fitting clothes made with natural fibres, such as cotton, and avoiding wool, silk and synthetic fabrics, which can tend to over-insulate, can be very helpful. Carrying excess weight can worsen hot flushes and weight loss can sometimes help. Planning your day to avoid last-minute rushing and stress can be really helpful to limit the flushes induced by being flustered.

For night-time symptoms similar principles apply. Keep your bedroom cool and avoid a hot bath or shower, or a hot drink, before bed. Light, cotton, breathable clothing is best, or sleep with light, cotton bed sheets only. Cooling pillows (infused with cooling gels and made with breathable fibres) or other cooling devices can be helpful for a few hours, earlier in the night.

Research data remains inconclusive in relation to the effects of exercise, yoga, controlled breathing, relaxation, meditation or other stress-reducing techniques in reducing hot flushes, but they do work for some people. They also help with other aspects of menopause, so they are worth a try. It is logical that if you are healthy and less stressed, the symptoms may feel less problematic.

Most evidence is insufficient, inconclusive or demonstrates no benefit for the use of herbs such as black cohosh, dong quai and evening primrose, and other supplements and techniques such as flaxseed, omega-3s, pollen extract, vitamin supplements, chiro-practic interventions and acupuncture in helping hot flushes. These herbs and supplements and techniques may sometimes help with other symptoms of menopause, so as long as they don't have any ill effects, they are fine to try out if you wish (see Chapter 13 for further information).

The main non-medication approach that has been shown to be effective in clinical trials is cognitive behavioural therapy (CBT). This is a psychological-based therapy that helps to challenge and change your unhelpful perceptions, thoughts and behaviours about symptoms, and can alter both the impact and severity of those symptoms. Studies looking at these approaches show a reduction in women's ratings of hot flush problems. You should be able to access CBT through your GP.

HRT appears the most effective treatment currently available for women with troubling menopausal hot flushes and sweats. Depending on individual risk assessment, HRT may provide justifiable benefits (see Chapter 15).

Non-hormone medications that have been shown to help with hot flushes and sweats include venlafaxine, paroxetine and fluoxetine. These are antidepressant medications but the dose required to help with hot flushes and sweats can be lower than the antidepressant dose. These options are recommended if you have severe sweats or hot flushes and choose not to have, or have risk factors for, HRT. These medications can improve your mood, help with sleep and improve flushes and sweats at low doses, so they are a useful option depending on your individual circumstances. In general, in low doses, these treatments appear to be well tolerated.

Clonidine is a medication that has been available for sweats and flushes for many decades. The reduction in sweating appears to be a beneficial side effect. If you do not want to take hormone treatment for your flushes and sweats, in particular if you have high blood pressure, clonidine is worth a try. It can also help with migraine. However, it can have side effects such as drowsiness, dizziness and low blood pressure and it doesn't suit everyone.

Oxybutynin is a medication used to treat an overactive bladder. It also seems to help with sweating so is sometimes used to ease these symptoms in menopause.

Gabapentin and pregabalin are strong medications that are more often used for chronic pain, but previously gained some research data in treating hot flushes and sweats. After concerns about addiction, however, and after a spike in the number of related deaths and a series of studies warning about the adverse effects of the medications, these drugs became 'Schedule 3' controlled drugs in the UK on 1 April 2019. I would not therefore recommend these drugs in menopause, nor did I before the change in policy.

As I have mentioned in previous chapters, a new treatment has recently been identified that may target the underlying hot flush mechanism in the brain and is currently undergoing advanced clinical trials. This could become a new safe alternative to HRT for relieving these and other menopause symptoms, but it is not yet licensed.

A quick recap

Hot flushes and night sweats are the most common symptom you are likely to experience during menopause. These symptoms usually settle over about two years but can last longer. Practical lifestyle measures can be very helpful to manage these symptoms. If you feel your symptoms are intolerable despite practical approaches, the choice of medication will depend on balancing your individual benefits and risks. You should be assisted in making treatment decisions by your supporting healthcare professionals.

CHAPTER 7

Managing Your Sleep

SLEEP DISRUPTION IS a common symptom through menopause. If you experience troublesome sleep problems these can have a knock-on effect on the rest of your life and can also affect your overall health, so this is another important lifestyle biohack to conquer. Difficulty getting to sleep, recurrent waking, not being able to get back to sleep, needing to empty your bladder, hot flushes, sweats, bed sheet changes, unexplained anxiety and palpitations are all very common.

Most people know that good-quality sleep is good for well-being. If you don't get enough sleep this can affect energy, focus, concentration, mood and motivation. What many people don't realise is that there appears to be even more to sleep than most of us are aware of.

A vast amount of research has been conducted into sleep in recent years, in particular looking at the negative health effects of 'short sleep duration'. This is defined as fewer than six hours' sleep per night. Short sleep has been found to be linked to an increased risk of diabetes, high blood pressure, heart diseases, obesity and overall risk of death. At the other end of the scale, too much sleep is also bad, although there has been less research into this problem.

A study published in 2019 in the *European Heart Journal* showed that both shorter (fewer than six hours per day) and longer (more than eight hours per day) estimated total sleep durations were associated with an increased risk of death and major heart and blood vessel problems (such as stroke, heart attacks or heart failure). The study concluded that a total sleep duration of six to eight hours per day is associated with the lowest risk of deaths and major heart attacks and strokes.

As menopause can worsen sleep quality and cause insomnia, does that mean if you have sleep disruption, you are at high risk of all those diseases listed above? The simple answer is no, because every single one of us is individual. A multitude of genetic and environmental factors contribute to your overall individual risk. There will, however, be some women whose health will suffer from sleep disruption through increased risk of heart and blood vessel diseases. It is therefore a win–win situation to optimise sleep, as this is likely to have a beneficial impact on your overall health and well-being.

MENOPAUSE NOW

There are many sleep disruptors that women going through menopause today are exposed to that were not around even a generation ago. These new issues, added to the well-recognised night sweats and flushes, racing heart and night-time anxiety, mean that sleep quality is more under threat than ever. Technology in the bedroom is a major newcomer in the top charts of sleep disruption in the last couple of decades. This links with excessive blue light screen exposure, which is discussed on page 88. But many other factors, including social stress, care roles, challenging jobs, deadlines, less physical activity, caffeine, alcohol, lack of lifestyle routine, excessive prescribed medications (many of which negatively affect

> sleep), lack of sunlight and jet lag, all play a role in fragmenting our sleep structure. All these factors have emerged for the first time, or become more intense, over the past few decades and are affecting society as a whole.

Rather than being disheartened by headlines about sleep, it is much better to focus on what proactive changes you can make to improve your sleep quality long-term. That's what I do as a self-confessed insomniac! It is logical that if you understand more about sleep you will be able to make choices to help improve your sleep quality and quantity.

I am going to talk a little bit about sleep in general before I go into the specific nuances of menopausal sleep disruption. Use the information and solutions to shape your sleep renewal.

SLEEP STAGES

During normal sleep, there are two distinct stages: REM (rapid eye movement) and NREM (non-rapid eye movement) sleep. NREM sleep is composed of four stages. On an average night there are five sleep cycles lasting around 90 minutes that involve all the stages of sleep starting with stage 1 NREM and ending with REM. Even if your sleep is disrupted, you will still go through the different sleep stages each night.

Each stage of sleep serves a unique restorative function, including muscle recovery, hormone regulation and memory consolidation, making it essential to allow enough time to cycle through all sleep stages. Without a full night of sleep, your body and mind are deprived of the essential elements needed to help you conquer the day.

Stage 1

This is known as the transitional phase. You float in and out of consciousness. You may be partially awake while you drift off. This is also the time when the muscles jerk, followed by a falling then jolt sensation (slip on a banana skin sensation). This phase usually lasts for 5–10 minutes. After winding down in Stage 1, you will slip into Stage 2.

Stage 2

Overall around half the time spent asleep over the course of the night is spent in Stage 2 sleep, and the amount of Stage 2 gets longer with each sleep cycle. The heart rate begins to slow and the core body temperature decreases. Muscle tone and muscle relaxation alternate.

Stages 3 and 4 (slow wave sleep)

These are deep stages of sleep, and are the hardest to wake up from. If you try to wake someone up when they are in Stages 3 or 4, they will most likely be disoriented and groggy for minutes after they wake. Stages 3 and 4 are often grouped together as 'deep sleep' because they are the periods of slow wave sleep. Most Stage 3 and 4 sleep occurs in the first part of your night's sleep. Stage 3 only lasts a few minutes and Stage 4 is longer, making up about 10–15 per cent of sleep time.

During slow wave sleep, blood pressure drops and breathing becomes deeper and slower. There is no eye movement, and the body becomes virtually paralysed. Blood flow to the muscles increases, providing them with restorative oxygen and nutrients. During these sleep stages, the body builds bone and strengthens the immune system. These are the stages when nightmares can occur.

Stages 3 and 4 of sleep are extremely rejuvenating and restorative to the body. Hormones are released that support both growth and appetite control. These hormones are essential to the maintenance of lean body mass and also help control overeating during the day.

REM sleep

This stage tends to happen at the end of each sleep cycle. The first period of REM typically lasts 10 minutes. Each of your later REM stages should get longer, and the final one may last up to an hour. There is therefore more REM sleep later in the night. Your heart rate and breathing quickens. You can have intense dreams during REM sleep, since your brain is more active. REM sleep is very restorative, and is when our bodies and minds undergo the most renewal.

Quality sleep is restorative to the nervous, skeletal and muscular systems. It helps maintain mood, memory and brain function, and plays a large role in the function of the hormone and immune systems.

As you get older, lighter stages of sleep tend to dominate and deep sleep can be lacking. You may also not need as much sleep as you get older.

ERROR 4.04 SLEEP NOT FOUND

Sleep is complex because there are different stages and multiple cycles each night, and even if you get enough overall sleep you may not wake refreshed if the sleep stages are not balanced. Frequent waking in menopause can be caused by many different factors including night sweats, needing to empty your bladder and sometimes for no obvious reason. Difficulty getting to sleep and early wakening are also common. Like with other aspects of menopause, this is an individual experience. What is certainly clear is that if your sleep feels disrupted, this can often affect your daytime well-being by causing fatigue, brain fog and needing to nap. These symptoms can put you off exercise if they make you feel drained and daytime fatigue can frequently make you reach for comfort food as an energy fix.

Although there are many factors that can disrupt sleep in menopause, night sweats and flushes seem to be the most common ones that women complain about. These do settle with time, but if they trigger a disrupted sleep habit, that can be difficult to break. There are also modern-day sleep disruptors unrelated directly to menopause that need attention from many of us and I will talk about them and provide some night-time hacks after sharing Jade's case history.

CASE HISTORY: JADE

Jade came to see me because she could not sleep. Her periods had stopped more than 12 months before and she knew she was menopausal but she didn't have many symptoms, except insomnia, which was resulting in daytime fatigue. She would wake up hot in the night, needing to empty her bladder, and would struggle to get back to sleep. These symptoms were disrupting Jade's job as an executive. She would sometimes lose her thread in work meetings and presentations due to brain fog. Jade had never had sleep problems before. She had never had to think about sleep routine and she did not realise that bad sleep habits can catch up with you in menopause.

Jade had always had a strong coffee in the evening just before clearing her work emails and then checking social media before jumping into bed, which could be any time between 10pm and 2am. She had done this for years and now suddenly she would be lying awake after jumping into bed instead of instantly dropping off as she had done all her life.

Jade had got away with poor sleep habits all her adult life, but menopause had arrived and was not cutting her any slack. Jade did not want to have HRT for her symptoms because she had a family history of breast cancer in several close female relatives.

Jade was very motivated to help herself get her sleep back on track, but she didn't know what to do. We discussed multiple sleep strategies, including sleep routine and sleep rituals, avoiding caffeine close to bedtime and the harmful effects of blue light screen exposure before bed. Jade implemented everything required. She did not notice an improvement at first, but she stuck at our plan, because she understood that sleep is complex and rebalancing her sleep stages and cycles would probably be a slow process. Slowly but surely her sleep improved back to an excellent level. Jade was happy with her new sleep schedule and felt that her daytime energy was better than it had been for years, probably because her poor sleep habits had been affecting her even before menopause by reducing her restorative sleep.

Good sleep hygiene

There are many simple sleep biohacks that, when combined, can improve your sleep quality gradually. But sleep patterns are habit-forming and can be challenging to alter, so to change a bad sleep pattern takes persistence. Here are some tips to get you started with improving your sleep in menopause:

- Try to keep to a regular sleep routine. Go to sleep and get up at a similar time each day. This supports a healthy sleep–wake cycle.

- Try to avoid daytime napping and, if you do nap, keep it short and ensure you don't do this in the late afternoon or evening. Fatigue related to disrupted night-time sleep can bring on 'sleep pressure' during the day, which is a desire or need to sleep and which can tempt you to take a nap if you have the opportunity. If you do this your body can get confused. The wakeful hormones can then kick in and keep you awake later that night.
- Do not drink caffeinated drinks after a certain point, especially if you are sensitive to them. Ideally have your last caffeine exposure in the early to mid-afternoon. It is not necessary for most people to cut out caffeine altogether. Decaffeinated drinks are an alternative, but these contain a lot of chemicals instead of caffeine.
- Exercise is great for health, but try not to do this too close to bedtime as it can cause a surge in adrenal and other hormones that can induce wakefulness.
- Try to avoid eating large meals too close to bedtime as the metabolic activity of your gut trying to empty your stomach, coupled with the risk of indigestion, can negatively affect the onset of sleep. Ideally leave two to three hours between a main meal and going to bed.
- Alcohol will not help sleep in a positive way. I am not saying don't drink alcohol, but certainly don't be misled into thinking it is helping you sleep. That is simply not correct.
- Alcohol and caffeinated drinks are also diuretics and make you pass more urine, so may worsen sleep disruption from needing to go to the toilet in the night. Excessive intake of any fluids in the hours close to bed can do this so, if you have to get up in the night to pee a lot, try to reduce alcohol and all drinks for two to three hours before bed. Regular practice of pelvic floor exercises can also help with needing to pee frequently at night (see page 51).

Night-time sleep hacks

- Try to keep a regular wind-down to sleep or 'sleep ritual'. This helps your body to anticipate sleep. This is broadly known as classical or Pavlovian conditioning. It doesn't have to be complicated. Some people read a book, listen to soothing music or soak in a warm bath. If you just stop what you're doing and go straight to bed, you have not allowed any wind-down time; your brain is likely to still be very active, full of thoughts from the day's activities and may be unable to fall asleep. Sleep rituals not only prepare you for sleep, but enable your brain to associate certain activities with sleep. Remember any new routine will take time for your body to 'acclimatise' to.

- Try to keep your bedroom uncluttered and keep it ring-fenced for relaxation and sleep. Try to avoid bringing any work- or stress-related equipment into the bedroom.

- If you take a warm or tepid shower or bath before bed, your body and mind may feel more tired afterwards, as it associates the shower with sleep. The fall in body temperature afterwards also helps with sleep onset.

- If possible use blackout curtains or blinds to reduce visual stimulation, which can keep you awake after lights out, or wake you up.

- If you have ever had a spa treatment you will recall the calming music and subtle scents that help relax you and often make you feel sleepy. This is an excellent model for winding down in the bedroom before sleep. Aromatherapy scents and meditative music or sounds during the time before lights out are easy to bring into the bedroom (swap phones and laptops for these). They will create an atmosphere of calm and relaxation.

- Sleeping pills only work when you take them, if at all, and can cause rebound insomnia when you stop them. They are therefore almost NEVER an effective solution to the sleep disruption of menopause.

Managing night sweats

To help reduce night sweats, avoid hot baths, showers or hot drinks before bed, wear light cotton, breathable clothing or de-clothe and use light cotton bed sheets with low thread counts and not too many layers. Ideally keep your bedroom on the cool side, which may mean turning the radiator off or opening a window depending on the weather. Use blankets that you can throw off when a flush or sweat arrives. Have a spare set of night clothes and bed sheets nearby in case a quick night change is needed. The use of cooling pillows (pillow gel mats and pillows infused with cooling gels and made with breathable fibres) and other cooling devices can be helpful.

HRT (see Chapter 15) helps with sleep quality and night sweats along with many other menopause symptoms. HRT frequently helps with but does not always resolve menopause sleep disruption, so it should be used in conjunction with other healthy sleep practices.

A new treatment is being developed, but is not yet available, that appears to help significantly with night sweats and sleep – watch this space.

Blue light exposure

You may not be aware that shutting off all electric devices for an hour or two before bedtime will help with sleep onset and quality. This includes watching TV and using mobile phones, laptops and electrical reading devices. The instant logic is that these devices keep your mind active and stimulated, perhaps driving up stress hormones due to the stressful content of the activity, whatever it is (e.g. a stressful work email or watching the news!). The adrenal stress hormones are closely linked with circadian rhythm. They have diurnal pulses, and can also pulse multiple times during a 24-hour period. High stress hormones at bedtime can cause insomnia.

Blue light exposure is emitted from screens, fluorescent and LED lights and can delay the release of sleep-inducing melatonin, increase alertness and reset the body's internal clock (or circadian rhythm) to a later schedule.

Although it is environmentally friendly, blue light can affect your sleep and potentially cause disease. Until the advent of artificial lighting, the sun was the major source of all lighting. The first electric light was invented in the early 1800s, only a couple of hundred years ago. Before that, people spent their evenings in relative darkness. It is only in the last few decades that the entire world has become globalised and there are now few places where night-time is reliably dark. Evenings are now brightly illuminated for most of us right until the point our head hits the pillow. This fundamental change is brilliant for allowing us to fit so much more activity into our day and to be more productive, but it also has some sinister effects. At night, light throws our body clock (the circadian rhythm) out of synch with health effects beyond sleep disruption. Misaligned body clocks are associated with an increased risk of high blood pressure, diabetes and prediabetes, among other health problems.

Not all colours of light have the same stimulating effect. Blue wavelengths, which are beneficial during daylight hours because they boost attention, reaction times and mood, seem to be the most disruptive at night. And the proliferation of electronics with screens, as well as energy-efficient LED lighting, is increasing our exposure to blue wavelengths, especially after sunset.

TVs, computers, laptops, smartphones, tablets, and fluorescent and LED lighting are all sources of blue light. When it comes to technology in the bedroom, you may well be sleeping with the enemy.

We know that daylight keeps an individual's body clock aligned with the environment. We also know that exposure to light suppresses the secretion of melatonin, a hormone that rises during sleep and follows a circadian rhythm.

While light of any kind can suppress the secretion of melatonin, blue light at night does so more powerfully than green or red light. Research studies have suggested that blue light suppresses melatonin for about twice as long as green light and shifts circadian rhythms by twice as much (three hours versus one-and-a-half hours). Studies suggest that of all synthetic light, dim red night lights are the least disruptive to sleep and may help improve mood. Red light has the least power to shift circadian rhythm and suppress melatonin, and has significantly less evidence of brain changes linked to depression when compared with blue light. But it is clear that total darkness at bedtime is best for sleep.

All electronic devices produce blue light and the evidence suggests exposure to these at bedtime worsens sleep quality. So, if you have insomnia, regardless of whatever else you address to help you sleep in menopause, even using HRT, if you are on your phone or tablet device close to bedtime you may not manage to achieve refreshing quality sleep. Sleep will be helped by avoiding looking at bright screens for two to three hours before bed. If you work a night shift or use a lot of electronic devices at night, consider wearing blue-blocking glasses or installing an app that filters the blue/green wavelength at night.

Mindful breathing

If you are unable to get to sleep or if you wake up sweaty and anxious with a flush, sweat or with your heart racing and then cannot get back to sleep, it's helpful to know what you can do to help induce sleep in the moment. It is very frustrating feeling desperate to sleep but unable to, and your anxiety can make this worse. In this situation try to focus on the fact that you are resting quietly and that is good for you in the context of your busy life, even though sleep would be better. In this situation, it can also be very helpful to learn and implement a type of brain training known as 'mindful breathing'.

Basic mindful breathing is not difficult to learn. It simply involves focusing your attention on your breath: breath in (inhalation) and breath out (exhalation). Ideally you should be lying in a comfortable position at a cool temperature. Your eyes may be open or closed, but you may find it easier to focus with them closed. Experts believe a regular practice of mindful breathing can make it easier for it to succeed in difficult situations, so if you can also find the time to do this intermittently during the day, that could help it to work when you are lying awake at night.

You can start by taking exaggerated breaths, first a deep breath in through the nostrils for three seconds, then hold your breath for four seconds and then breathe out through your mouth for five seconds. You can adjust the number of seconds in each phase to work for you. They are not fixed. You can alternatively simply observe each breath without trying to adjust it; it may help to focus on the rise and fall of your chest or the sensation through your nostrils. As you do so, you may find that your mind wanders, distracted by thoughts or sensations. That is fine, but you need to acknowledge and notice that this is happening and gently bring your attention back to your breath. These simple steps can help encourage sleep at these difficult points in the night.

MINDFUL BREATHING TO HELP IN THE MOMENT

- Make yourself comfortable.
- Breathe in through your nose for three counts.
- Hold at the top of your breath for four counts.
- Exhale through your mouth for five counts.
- Repeat the process.
- Try to let go of all your negative thoughts and feelings with your breath out.

A word about bed partners

Many of us sleep with a partner, some of whom will sleep well, some not so well and others may suffer insomnia. The arrival of a new sleep disturbance in menopause can affect our partners too. Shared thinking and mutual understanding can be helpful.

How you make that adjustment will be different for everyone. For example, trying to make sure the bedroom temperature is cool is a simple step. Your partner may need to wrap up warm! If you are easily woken, it will be really important for your partner to avoid making noise when they come to bed if you are already asleep. Ideally your partner should not be on their phone or watching TV in the bedroom if you are trying to sleep. There should be no smoking in the bedroom. Snoring issues can worsen insomnia and some couples may have the option to sleep separately sometimes for the sake of a better night's sleep. Solutions will be unique to each couple. If you have kids, it can sometimes be helpful to think back to those newborn days and whether any adjustments you made then could be rejigged to minimise sleep disruption for both parties today. If not, you may need to go back to the drawing board.

STRATEGIES TO OPTIMISE SLEEP

I have listed below all of the sleep hacks that will be helpful for your overall sleep quality. The more strategies that you are able to apply, the more likely your sleep will revert gradually to a healthy balance between sleep stages and cycles.

- Set a sleep routine and keep it consistent.
- Avoid or limit daytime naps.
- No caffeine past late afternoon.
- Limit fluid intake and alcohol before bed.
- Keep your bedroom uncluttered.
- Maintain a cool bedroom temperature.
- Avoid a hot shower, bath or hot drink at bedtime.
- Use blackout curtains or blinds.
- Try soothing scents and sounds.

- Wear light cotton, breathable clothing or de-clothe and use light cotton bed sheets.
- Have a spare set of night clothes nearby in case a quick night change is needed.
- Avoid sleeping pills.
- Dump those electronic devices outside the room.
- Use a dim red night light if needed.
- Try to practise mindful breathing exercises if you find yourself awake, anxious and unable to sleep.

A quick recap

Sleep is a very important daily event and getting it right is vital for your overall health and well-being during menopause. Knowledge about sleep and sleep disruptors will hopefully help to motivate you to make the modest changes needed to improve your sleep in the long term.

Sleep hacks can make a big difference because they can help you with all aspects of sleep quality, including modern-day sleep issues, that can worsen your menopause sleep problems. Achieving a good sleep pattern through menopause needs attention to detail because lots of different factors can be contributing and the solutions take time to work, so perseverance with good sleep habits is all-important.

Weight Management

ALMOST ALL WOMEN going through menopause notice a change in body shape and fat distribution (it goes on the tummy). You may notice that your weight is much more difficult to keep under control, even if you take HRT. This is because of changes in your metabolism (see pages 99–100). You are likely to be very motivated to keep your weight healthy and doing so reduces the risk of many health problems. Weight management is not only important for how you feel about yourself, but also for your long-term health. Keeping a healthy weight is for life, not just for after Christmas!

WHAT IS A HEALTHY WEIGHT?

It is important for your overall health to keep a healthy weight after menopause, but what does this look like? Doctors usually use body mass index (BMI) to assess weight because it measures your weight in proportion to your height and this gives a better estimation of whether your weight is on-target for health, or not. BMI is a useful measure that has been used in many studies of health risk, but it is not perfect. Some people who are very muscular or who have heavy bones may appear overweight when they actually have normal body fat but high muscle or bone density. The opposite can apply for people who are of normal BMI.

You can calculate your own BMI using your weight and height with an online calculator. Or you can have a look at the following NHS chart to see if you are the right weight based on your height:

HEIGHT/WEIGHT CHART

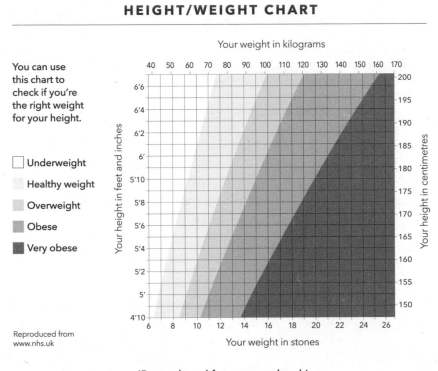

(Reproduced from www.nhs.uk)

Being either underweight or obese can be associated with health problems. Recent research suggests that, for most people, being borderline overweight may be an advantage as you get older, but a BMI of over 30 appears to increase the risk of some cancers and other diseases. The risk for those diseases appears to increase further as BMI rises. It is therefore helpful to know which category you are in.

In the table below I have listed the different BMI categories and described any health risks or benefits associated with each category. Once you've calculated your BMI, you can look at any health risks that your BMI category may carry. Risks do not mean you are guaranteed to get those problems, but it allows you to understand whether a change in your weight could help your overall health.

BMI categories and associated health risks

BMI (kg/m²)	Category	Health risks after menopause
Less than 18	Underweight	Weakened immune system, fragile bones and feeling tired
18–25	Normal	Reduced risk of heart disease, stroke, several cancers, type 2 diabetes, back and joint problems, and osteoporosis, and better immune function
25–27	Borderline	Some studies suggest this is the lowest risk of death from any cause and may be the most favourable category for older women, even though it was previously classed as overweight
27–30	Overweight	Increased risk of heart and blood vessel disease, gallbladder disease, high blood pressure, type 2 diabetes, osteoarthritis, certain types of cancer, such as colon and breast cancer, depression and other mental health disorders

BMI (kg/m²)	Category	Health risks after menopause
30–35	Moderately obese	Further increased risk of heart and blood vessel disease, gallbladder disease, high blood pressure, type 2 diabetes, osteoarthritis, certain types of cancer, such as colon and breast cancer, depression and other mental health disorders
35–44	Severely obese	Further increased risk of heart and blood vessel disease, gallbladder disease, high blood pressure, type 2 diabetes, osteoarthritis, certain types of cancer, such as colon and breast cancer, depression and other mental health disorders
45–50	Morbidly obese	Further increased risk of heart and blood vessel disease, gallbladder disease, high blood pressure, type 2 diabetes, osteoarthritis, certain types of cancer, such as colon and breast cancer, depression and other mental health disorders
Greater than 50	Super obese	Highest risk of heart and blood vessel disease, gallbladder disease, high blood pressure, type 2 diabetes, osteoarthritis, certain types of cancer, such as colon and breast cancer, depression and other mental health disorders

Our weight affects how we feel about ourselves. If your weight is under control and you are happy with it, you will feel better and more confident. It is a good idea to try to decide realistically where you want your weight and BMI to be so that you can work towards your goal, or maintain it if you are already there.

In this chapter I want to provide some insight about why the weight of the whole of the Western world is increasing and how you, as an individual, can defy this trend, despite menopause. In our twenty-first-century world, instincts will often trick us into thinking we are hungry when desirable food is calling us and is available. Eating can be a habit that is easy to inadvertently overdo. You may also comfort eat if you feel stressed or tired, but you may not really need to eat at that time. When metabolism dips in menopause these habits and instincts can cause weight gain. Heading into menopause is therefore a good opportunity to refocus on weight management.

WHAT IS METABOLISM?

Metabolism is a term used to describe the sum total of chemical reactions in the body's cells that change food into energy. It effectively measures the rate at which the body converts stored energy into working energy.

There are many hormones and chemicals that contribute to metabolism, but one of the very important metabolic hormones is insulin. Insulin regulates how the body uses and stores sugar, fat and protein from food. If you have a meal rich in calories these need to be stored quickly and efficiently with the help of insulin, to stop the blood filling up with sugar or fat and causing diabetes.

Insulin resistance

Insulin resistance is a metabolic problem in which muscle, fat and liver cells start resisting or ignoring insulin signals. More insulin is needed to achieve the goal of getting sugar out of the bloodstream and into cells.

There are genetic factors that predispose some people to insulin resistance, but too much tummy fat is a common cause in the Western world. Insulin resistance is also linked to other lifestyle factors including lack of exercise, smoking and insufficient sleep. As insulin resistance develops, your body fights back by producing more insulin and this can trigger prediabetes. This is associated with high blood pressure and high cholesterol. These conditions can predispose to type 2 diabetes.

Menopause and advancing age are both linked with insulin resistance, a fall in metabolic rate and a shift to increased tummy fat. The lower your metabolic rate the easier it can be to gain weight.

But you have choices. Increased muscle bulk from exercise can increase your metabolic rate. Being knowledgeable and mindful about the changes in your metabolism through menopause will enable you to be discerning with the choices you make. Limiting weight gain or shedding excess weight and maintaining physical activity and strengthening your muscles through menopause will boost your metabolism. These choices will also have a positive impact on well-being and health, as well as weight balance through menopause.

MENOPAUSE NOW

Our female ancestors were susceptible to disease and starvation. If the family could not provide food for them, menopause was a dangerous state. Because of this genetic baggage, meant to be protective, our metabolism is naturally switched to calorie preservation in menopause. Our environment in the Western world is very different now. Understanding this is important because frequent dietary indiscretions and consumption of 'empty calories' can be a contributor to weight gain in menopause, when it would not necessarily have had the same effect before menopause.

Understanding menopause metabolism

I have heard the following expression from my patients many times: 'I have always eaten the same, but now my weight is rising for no reason.' When you consider the impact of changing hormones on your metabolism, it is logical that a lower metabolism in menopause means you don't need as many calories to keep the same weight.

Eating in the same way as you did in your younger years can therefore result in seemingly unexplained weight gain as you get older. This is because your metabolism has shifted downwards, so eating the same equates to calorie input now exceeding calorie expenditure.

Eating slightly surplus to requirements over a number of years can result initially in minor weight gain. During a busy life, it is very easy for gradual weight gain to go unnoticed. Unless weight becomes noticeably above target, this issue may not be on your radar. If weight does become a noticeable problem, it will race to the top of your priority list, and the mindset to take action is triggered. For those of you reading this who are of normal weight, prevention is better than cure. If your weight is fine at the moment, read on to keep it that way.

MY WEIGHT MANAGEMENT STORY

I am often described as petite. When I am advising my patients about weight management many say to me, 'Well it's easy for you because you are naturally slim.' And I am thinking, 'Oh no I am not!' So then I tell them my story because you cannot judge a book by its cover.

We know that genes have a major role in weight balance and metabolism, and some people are naturally built thin, while others will always tend to gain weight easily. My wonderful eighty-year-old mum struggled with her weight from her early forties after stopping smoking and has been overweight ever since. My dear late father, who was from India, had the genes that put all his weight on his middle so he had a big tummy. Essentially, my genes would suggest I should now (in menopause) be overweight. The reason I am not is because, as a doctor, I have always been careful with unhealthy foods and conscious about the health implications of weight balance. Studying diabetes and endocrinology as a post-graduate doctor for the last 25 years has helped me to understand the changes in foods available that has driven the diabetes epidemic and it has influenced my own eating behaviours in a positive way. It has made me more mindful about food. I have also been mindful about my metabolism dipping in menopause and so to counteract that I ensure I do as much exercise as I can to burn off my guilty pleasures (generally chocolate and fizzy wine). I am not perfect (none of us are), but I am not slim because I was built to be – it is the product of knowledge, mindfulness and commitment. And that's why I wanted to include this chapter – to share my knowledge with you and help to inform and empower you to do the same.

HOW TO LOSE WEIGHT SUSTAINABLY

Rapid, short-term weight-loss diets use a variety of different approaches, including weight management support groups and very low-calorie diets. These can appear attractive and, in the early days, be effective in shedding the pounds. We know that very low-calorie diets can work in the short term. However, keeping the weight off in the long term is much more challenging. It is not easy to shed several years of gradual weight gain in a few weeks of extreme calorie restriction, especially in menopause.

Most of these short-term diets and weight-loss interventions typically result in early rapid weight loss of varying degrees, followed by a weight plateau and then gradual weight regain. Extreme calorie restriction also causes hunger and fatigue, and is therefore difficult to sustain for long enough to make extreme diets work in the long term. Seeing poor results from an extreme diet can be disheartening. It is then easy to quit your efforts and regain the lost weight.

Gradual weight reduction approaches, using a combination of lifestyle measures, including increased calorie burning through exercise, stress reduction, choosing more nutritious food options and being mindful about the impact of occasional binge eating as well as the calorie load from alcohol and other drinks, are likely to be effective and sustainable approaches in shedding the excess weight long-term. There are many tricks and skills you can apply to help limit calorie intake without it feeling extreme or making you feel too restricted. Choosing strategies that you feel are doable for you and sticking to them will enable them to become engrained and fit in to your routine.

Remember one size does not fit all and sustained results are not usually dramatic, sudden or striking in the short term. This means that your mindset and expectations need to be tempered. There are some common themes that help weight loss so let's start with those. There are some obvious, and some not so obvious, do's and don'ts:

- Try not to keep guilty pleasures in the house readily available for moments of weakness.
- Only shop for what you need that week and do not stockpile food that may be consumed too quickly in a moment of weakness.
- Don't go food shopping when you are hungry – you will generally buy more than you need!
- If you need a snack in between meals try to avoid unhealthy options such as crisps, biscuits, chocolate and any other

processed fast food option. Keep a fruit bowl to pick from or snack on nuts, seeds, vegetable sticks (cucumber, carrot, pepper, celery, etc.), which you can pre-prepare and keep ready in your fridge.

- If you drive a lot, only keep healthy snack options in your car.
- If you feel thirsty, drink water rather than fizzy drinks or other drinks with empty calories.
- Be mindful that drinks other than water may contain a lot of calories. A large glass (250ml) of average strength wine contains about 200 calories. One shot of vodka or gin has approximately one quarter of the calories if consumed with low-calorie tonic. Beware the regular coffee catch-up with friends: a single full-fat cappuccino is roughly 165 calories, while a skinny cappuccino is 96 calories.

Transform the way you feel

It is much easier to lose weight when you feel well and have good energy levels and are not stressed. If you are exhausted, the added fatigue induced by low blood sugar, brought on by calorie restriction, is unlikely to be sustainable. For these reasons, it is important to try to address, as best as possible, any of these lifestyle or health issues before putting added pressure on yourself to lose weight. When women in menopause feel stressed and exhausted, they are also likely to do less activity and comfort eat. In this situation, it will be easy to gain weight. My recommendation in this situation is to address the underlying issues affecting your well-being first and foremost, and simply aim to keep your weight stable during this period. Once you start to feel better, greater focus on weight loss will be more achievable. You will find helpful solutions about improving well-being through approaches to exercise (Chapter 4), nutrition (Chapter 5), sleep (Chapter 7), managing fatigue (Chapter 11) and stress management (Chapters 9 and 10), which make up the other menopause toolkit sections of this book. All the tricks and lifestyle tweaks in those chapters will improve and transform how you feel and you will be more able to stick to healthy eating and calorie restriction if needed.

Get moving

For the vast majority of women in menopause, the most effective way to keep a healthy weight or achieve long-term weight loss is through sustainable lifestyle approaches. The first and most important measure to implement is physical activity.

Regular daily activity will increase calorie burn – a 30-minute walk every day, over and above your usual daily routine, will burn approximately 150 calories for a woman around menopause. This is an estimate, but if you can do that every day you will burn an extra 1,050 or so calories per week. That is enough to counteract the effect of the occasional guilty pleasure and can help to keep your weight steady.

Small measures, such as taking the stairs instead of using a lift, or parking the car or getting off public transport a bit further away from your destination to allow you to do some extra walking, are profoundly effective in helping with weight management in the long term and aren't too hard to dovetail into your routine. Any movement is better than no movement. Even five minutes' walking is time well spent and will burn calories. Small steps such as these are also helpful for many other aspects of well-being. After a successful exercise session the happy hormones (endorphins) will be released, stress hormones will be regulated, pain will be kept in check and mood boosted. And lowering stress hormones also helps with weight loss. (See Chapter 4 for lots more advice on building exercise into your daily routine.)

Beware the empty calories

Ditching empty calories – such as the odd packet of crisps, or the odd biscuit or cake – wherever possible can make a notice-able difference to weight management. If you don't have these regularly your mind will tell you that the odd one will do no harm. However, though the odd one will make a tiny difference, the odd one again and again over weeks, months and years accumulates on the waistline. Therefore, using a mindful approach to eating can make a tremendous difference to weight management without really even feeling like you are restricting. For example, in between meals if you reach for a snack, consider asking yourself whether you really need it. When you have a meal, eating on the go and rushing food can result in eating more than if you sit down to eat without distraction and eat your meal more slowly.

Awareness of these considerations is important. Little changes, such as having a glass or two less of wine at the weekends, and having one or two alcohol-free days during the week, can make a big positive long-term difference to your overall health and weight management.

When you want to reach for the odd guilty pleasure, or the extra course of a meal when you are already feeling full, think waistline, and think about whether that indulgence is really necessary or worth it. If you consciously think about it in a mindful way, you will probably decide to pass on the indulgence at least some of the time. That will have a positive result over months and years, and will manifest as a noticeable improvement on your waistline.

TOP TIP: A JUSTIFIED TREAT

Dark chocolate, which is high in cocoa solids (70–80 per cent), has a higher content (compared with milk chocolate) of cocoa flavanols and fibre, which have health benefits. If chocolate is your foible, choosing dark chocolate over milk chocolate appears to have some health benefits.

Keep track of progress

Measuring your weight regularly and keeping a general track of calorie intake is helpful for weight loss in menopause for most women. Keeping a food diary is a really useful way of keeping track of what you're consuming, and can help you eat fewer calories and lose weight. It is so easy to inadvertently consume more calories than you are expending and eat slightly beyond your needs, even if you think you are being good. For example, even if you eat super-healthy food, inadvertently large portion sizes can still contribute to weight gain. If you are mindful and monitor your food intake and weight regularly, it can be easier to keep weight in check in the longer term. If you do not have any weight management concerns then this will not be relevant to you.

Practise portion control

Practising portion control is very important. With any type of dietary approach, no matter how healthy and balanced, you need to keep in mind that if you eat too many calories overall, beyond your metabolic need, you'll gain weight. Even nutritious, low-fat, plant-based foods, if eaten in a large enough quantity, can cause weight gain. So, if you think you are eating healthily but your weight is going up, you will need to cut down your portion sizes.

Eat mindfully

You know you need to be careful with calories, but you still have to live and thrive. You don't need to restrict excessively – the key here is mindful eating and moderation. You must be enabled to splice some guilty pleasures and treats into your eating schedule, and that is fine as long as you try to balance any indulgences with moderating calorie intake at other times or burning off those extra calories through exercise to keep your weight steady. Being mindful at each mealtime is also very helpful – simply not rushing your meal and focusing while eating will reduce the likelihood of inadvertent overindulgence. Also, the appetite hormones that tell you that you are full don't have time to work if you eat too quickly, so eating slowly and mindfully will allow your appetite centre to tell you that you are full at the right time.

MENOPAUSE NOW

Even 50 years ago the types of food available to buy were totally different than they are today. Ready meals, processed and fast food, takeaway meals and eating out in restaurants were all rarities. Now these types of food and eating styles are the norm in the Western world.

THE TRUTH ABOUT PROCESSED FOOD

Processed food is food that has been modified in some way mechanically or chemically to change its nature or preserve it. Foods can go through various levels of processing. Many processed foods are labelled to appear appealing by having some apparent health advantage. Beware that this may be fake news.

Processed foods are designed to taste good so that you will keep buying them. This often means that they contain large amounts of fat, sugar and salt, though the labelling rarely makes this clear. Examples include ready-prepared cooking sauces, ready meals, pizzas, oven chips, pies and most takeaway food.

While processed foods are high in fat, sugar and protein, they are also usually low in micronutrients – the vitamins and minerals that we cannot make in our body and which we obtain from food (see page 60). Vitamins and minerals are the building blocks of well-being and are essential for many aspects of menopause health. Processed foods are also usually low in fibre and need to have an extended shelf life, so they frequently contain chemical preservatives. Reading food labels is a really useful exercise to develop an understanding of how much sugar and fat as well as chemicals are in these foods. The marketing of processed foods can make unbalanced products appear healthy.

The truth is, and this is now very clear from many independent investigations, that many processed foods are actually driving the obesity and diabetes epidemics in the Western world because they are so unbalanced. The same principles apply to sugary drinks. Fizzy drinks and concentrated fruit juices contain alarming amounts of sugar. Some energy drinks can amount to a meal's worth of calories and can spike blood sugar. Sugar-free fizzy drinks contain chemicals that could be carcinogenic, instead of sugar. These artificial drinks, whether they contain sugar, or sugar substitutes, are very processed and not good for overall health.

It is not difficult to reduce or remove these foods and drinks from your diet if you have the right mindset. This is about thinking differently and stocking your kitchen in a different way. Natural food does not need to be expensive or time-consuming to prepare. Stock up with fresh fruit and vegetables – rainbow colours give you a good balance – and eggs, chickpeas, lentils, nuts and seeds. Experiment with fresh fruit smoothies if you have a smoothie maker (you can also use frozen fruit) and add chia seeds, carrots and spinach to these for extra fibre and micronutrients. Have a piece of fruit instead of a concentrated fruit juice drink and drink plenty of water. Scrambled eggs, omelettes, baked potatoes and home-made soups are examples of easy, quick on-the-go meals. You can make ratatouille and risottos with your favourite ingredients, and casseroles can be made in advance and filled with lots of plant-based ingredients and your choice of protein. (See also Chapter 8 and Appendix 2 for more useful tips.)

Wheat belly

There is one type of processed food that is so ubiquitous that we sometimes don't even consider it as processed – and that is refined wheat-based food. A thousand years ago wheat grain was a life-saving crop and bread was a staple carbohydrate and protein food source. Even today when eaten as the whole grain, wheat is a source of multiple nutrients and dietary fibre. Global demand for wheat is increasing due to the unique properties of gluten proteins, which facilitate the production of many processed foods. Wheat-based foods include bread, pasta, cakes, biscuits, pastry and pizza. These foods are usually not eaten in the whole grain form. Fibre and micronutrients are extracted in many cases, leaving a high quantity of concentrated calories. Eating a lot of this type of wheat-based food can therefore inadvertently contribute to weight gain, while cutting it down can have the opposite effect.

It's therefore important to think about how you can modify your wheat intake. You don't have to cut it out completely, unless you are coeliac or significantly gluten intolerant. Wholegrain wheat options are much better for health. Other good sources of carbs include: brown rice, nuts, seeds, potato with skin, sweet potato, vegetables, salad leaves, fruit, lentils, pulses, quinoa, oats, and more. None of these foods are significantly processed. They contain slow-release carbs and, in many cases, will be rich in micronutrients and fibre. These carb sources are likely to be good for overall well-being and weight management.

KEY FACT

A word of caution: 'gluten-free' processed foods appear to be just as processed as processed wheat itself and may contain many chemicals. Turning to gluten-free bread, pasta and so on is not usually therefore a healthier alternative to wheat. Unprocessed forms of wheat, for example wholewheat flour and wheat bran, have beneficial health effects and should not be classed as bad food choices. Unprocessed forms of wheat are absolutely fine as long as you are not coeliac (allergic to gluten). When you do have wheat try to have it in whole grain form.

CASE HISTORY: JENNY

Jenny came to see me in clinic complaining of weight gain. She was 48 years old and very physically active. She also had a busy stressful job but thought she had a very healthy diet and felt that the calories she was consuming must be less than her calorie burn.

Jenny was perimenopausal and her metabolism was changing. She was quite stressed with her job, and stress can hinder weight loss. Jenny's food diary showed that she was consuming energy drinks (labelled as healthy) that were high in sugar, and she was sometimes using these as meal substitutes. She always had breakfast, which was fruit, yoghurt with extra fresh fruit or a cereal bar. Jenny would have a couple of glasses of wine every night to de-stress. The rest of her diet was very healthy.

On the face of it Jenny should not be gaining weight. But her menopause metabolism was very sensitive to sugar and her body was responding to the sugar in the energy drinks, cereal bars, natural yoghurt and wine by producing extra insulin to store calories and block fat-burning.

Jenny did not know that the yoghurt she was having was full of sugar. As it was labelled 'fat-free' she thought it was healthy, but the reality was it actually contained more than 90 per cent rapid-release sugars. She also didn't realise the energy drinks and wine were so high in sugar and calories. These high-sugar foods can also cause sugar crashes and hunger a few hours after eating them, so Jenny was sometimes eating extra snacks and thought that her hunger and fatigue at those times were due to her exercise. She was actually having sugar crashes due to the refined sugar she was inadvertently consuming.

All Jenny had to do was ditch the energy drinks, cereal bars and yoghurt. She cut out the wine on a couple of nights per week and switched to natural, unprocessed meals and snacks. She was very careful to read food labels to identify whether foods dressed up to look healthy were actually high in sugar and therefore not good for a menopause metabolism.

Jenny gradually started to lose the weight that had been accumulating. Her exercise was maintained and she felt better because the sugar rush and crash sensations disappeared once the processed food was eradicated.

Deciphering sugar in food

Many processed foods contain sugar even when they don't taste sweet. Several processed foods and snacks labelled 'low-fat' can be high in sugar. For example, cereal bars marketed as convenient, on-the-go breakfast substitutes can be very high in sugar. Natural yoghurt is promoted as low-fat and high in calcium. This is true, but it can also be high in sugar. Many people (like Jenny in the above example) who are trying to watch their weight see the label 'low-fat' and believe that it must be a healthy option for weight loss, but some fruit yoghurts that are marketed as healthy can have as much as 15.8g of sugar per serving. That is almost 4tsp of sugar!

If you look on packaged and processed food labels you will see a summary of the quantity of sugar, fat, protein and salt. Some, but not all, will have traffic light colour codes to demonstrate if the food is high in sugar or fat.

If you look at the sugar content in grams on food packaging you can work out how many teaspoons of sugar are in that food by using the table below.

Teaspoon to grams of sugar conversion

Teaspoon	Grams
1tsp granulated sugar	4g sugar

Looking at food labels is helpful because you will see the total carbohydrate content and then a second comment 'of which sugars are'. The amount is usually given in grams (g). So, if a natural yoghurt says, 'per 120-g serving there are 16.3g carbs, of which 15.8g are sugar', that yoghurt contains almost 4tsp of sugar. Sugar is a fast-release carb, so this yoghurt is 97 per cent fast-release carbs, which can spike your blood sugar, and only contains about 3 per cent slow-release carbs, which are the good carbs. It therefore contains a lot of hidden sugar. Not all yoghurts will have such high amounts of sugar so it is important to read the label so that you can make the best choice for you.

Slow-release carbs

Not all carbohydrates release energy at the same rate (see page 58). Slow-release carbs are like a superfood. They do not spike your blood sugar and provide a slower and more sustained release of energy. They keep your appetite in check for longer than high-sugar foods and prop up energy levels and concentration through the day. They are also good for your heart and lower your cholesterol.

An example of a slow-release carb food is lentils. We know that 100g of lentils will contain approximately 20g of carbs, but only 1.8g of sugar i.e. 91 per cent slow-release carbs. Lentils also contain protein, vitamins and lots of dietary fibre. I describe foods like lentils as superfoods because they are all-round good guys.

Other natural slow-release carb foods also usually contain lots of vitamins, minerals and fibre and so have lots of health benefits (see Chapter 8). These include wholegrain cereals, vegetables, pulses, quinoa, nuts, seeds and many fresh fruits. The fewer processed foods you eat the more calories you will be able to obtain from healthy foods that are likely to contain more beneficial nutrients and keep you satisfied for longer.

The 'good' fats

For many years health guidelines urged us to restrict fat from our diets whenever possible because too much animal fat is known to raise cholesterol and is bad for the heart and blood vessels. We therefore switched to low-fat foods. But the shift didn't make us healthier, probably because we cut back on healthy fats as well as harmful ones. Your body needs some fat because it helps you absorb some vitamins and minerals. It is also important for blood clotting, muscle movement and inflammation, as well as being a major source of energy.

In recent years there has been a rise in processed foods made with artificial trans fats and other refined and highly processed oils. These processed fats now appear to be just as bad as or worse for the health than saturated animal fat. This has created confusion about what fat is good and what is bad.

We now know that good fats include monounsaturated and polyunsaturated fats. Bad ones include industrial-made processed trans fats. Saturated fats (from meat and dairy) fall somewhere in the middle.

We know that natural unsaturated fats, particularly as part of the Mediterranean diet, which typically includes lots of vegetables, fruits, whole grains, beans, nut and seeds, and olive oil, are very good for health and reduce the risk of many chronic diseases including heart disease. In essence, once again natural food with minimal processing is best. Too much animal fat and processed artificial fats both contain unnecessary calories that can worsen weight gain as well as having other negative health consequences.

CHOOSING AN APPROACH THAT'S RIGHT FOR YOU

If you want to reduce your weight you will need to choose an approach that works best for you to decrease your overall calorie intake. The best approach will be different for different people. Lowering your calorie intake to a level that can be sustained indefinitely, from week to week, is key.

Calorie-counting plans

If your routine does not change much day to day then sticking to a slightly reduced calorie plan every day is worth a try, and there are a number of brilliant smartphone applications that can calculate your energy intake and expenditure to guide you to sustained weight loss.

Time-restricted eating

If you don't have the time or inclination to input every consumed calorie into your phone app then there are other ways to achieve weight loss.

Another way to ensure a general modest calorie restriction is by having a long food-free zone on a daily basis – the so-called 'time-restricted approach' – for example, eating your last meal relatively early in the evening, to allow 12–16 hours until the next meal. A study published in the *Journal of Nutrition and Healthy Aging* in 2018 found that 8-hour time-restricted eating (i.e. having 16 hours of fasting) produced mild calorie restriction and weight loss, without calorie-counting. It also indicated possible clinical benefits by reducing blood pressure.

Intermittent fasting

If your routine is constantly changing it will be difficult for you to implement these fixed routine approaches. Another calorie-restriction method that has been growing in popularity in recent years is intermittent fasting, subtly different from time-restricted eating. It can be applied in different ways, but it does not really matter how it is done. It's the central principle and end result that matters.

If you like to go out, or eat and drink socially on certain days, restricting calorie intake on other days can help to maintain weight stability or achieve weight loss. The amount of intermittent restriction of calories balanced with the amount of intermittent calorie relapses will dictate whether weight stays stable or starts to fall, and you will need to monitor and adapt to what is needed. Regular weigh-ins are essential in guiding this approach.

If you skip a couple of meals, spaced out, once or twice a week, you may achieve an overall net negative calorie balance of anything from 1,000 to 2,000 calories per week, depending on your portion size and the types of food you are eating (see page 247 for more on this).

The metabolically attractive aspect of missing one meal occasionally is that you still have regular calories coming in on a daily basis, so your body doesn't notice the restriction as acutely as with an extreme diet. The body therefore seems to 'tolerate' the mild restriction better and facilitates, rather than blocks, the burning of fat. With this type of dietary approach, you may be restricting quite a lot overall from week to week, but in a less boom-and-bust way compared with extreme diets.

OTHER CAUSES OF WEIGHT GAIN

Weight-gain medications

As you get older it is easy to find yourself prescribed a number of medications for several different symptoms. There are several medications that can contribute to weight gain, so if you think a medication you are taking may be affecting your weight, consider discussing it with your GP to see if there is an alternative that you could change to that would be weight-neutral. Below is a list of some common medications that can cause weight gain and some treatments that can be used as an alternative. You will see that using alternatives is not always easy and should always be discussed with your GP.

Medications that can cause weight gain

Medication leading to weight gain	Alternative treatment options
Codeine, morphine, fentanyl, for pain	Paracetamol, non-steroidal pain drugs (NSAIDs), direct joint injections, treating the underlying cause of pain, physiotherapy, pain management programmes
Some antidepressants e.g. mirtazapine, amitriptyline, sertraline	Using psychological techniques for mood such as CBT. Some antidepressants do not cause weight gain
Mood regulators (neuroleptics), such as sulpiride, olanzapine, quetiapine, risperidone, haloperidol, lithium	Specialist psychiatric advice recommended
Gabapentin and pregabalin, for pain	Paracetamol, non-steroidal pain drugs (NSAIDs), direct joint injections, treating the underlying cause of pain, physiotherapy, pain management programmes

Medication leading to weight gain	Alternative treatment options
Steroids e.g. tablet prednisolone, injection methylprednisolone, injection kenalog, and high-dose inhaled steroids such as flixotide at doses of 1mg daily or more	Depends on the underlying medical problem. Some new immune treatments can be used instead of steroids and do not cause weight gain but can have a lot of other side effects
Some diabetes medications such as insulin and sulphonylureas	Using diabetes medications that do not cause weight gain where possible
Some blood pressure medications such as beta blockers	Several alternative blood pressure treatments do not cause weight gain
Antiepileptic medication such as valproate, carbamazepine, gabapentin	Specialist neurologist advice needed
Antihistamines	No real alternative currently but their effects are mild

Medical causes of weight gain

There are several medical conditions that can worsen weight difficulties and may occur in menopause. If you have any of these it is worth discussing with your doctor if there is anything additional that can be done to help with weight management.

- Underactive thyroid (hypothyroidism) is most commonly seen in women between the ages of 40 and 50 years. Symptoms of an underactive thyroid can overlap with menopausal symptoms. An underactive thyroid can therefore easily go unnoticed during the early stages of menopause.

- Adrenal and pituitary hormone gland problems, including Cushing's syndrome, can occur at any age and cause weight gain, but these are rare.
- Polycystic ovary syndrome (PCOS) is a condition that usually initially presents around puberty but can cause metabolic problems and weight gain around menopause.
- Diseases that lead to immobility due to chronic pain problems, such as inflammatory arthritis and fibromyalgia, can worsen and cause weight difficulties around menopause.

A quick recap

Many women are able to keep a healthy weight through menopause by making small changes to their eating patterns in conjunction with other lifestyle measures, such as increasing exercise and reducing fatigue and stress over time.

Even if you cut the bad stuff in your diet down by a fraction, and increase better-quality food by the same amount, that will have a positive impact on your health. You can then work towards further changes gradually over time if needed.

Mindfully choosing a dietary approach that suits your lifestyle, and being thoughtful about what you eat and when you eat it, will be liberating. This will help you conquer weight balance and improve your overall health lifelong.

CHAPTER 9

Understanding Stress

Sleep

S TRESS IS A physiological process in the human body that is meant to be protective. When imbalanced, stress can trigger anxiety and symptoms of anxiety can worsen the stress response. The stress burden of women going through menopause today means that they may be more susceptible to experiencing symptoms of anxiety. As anxiety is a psychological symptom of the stress response, reducing anxiety in menopause will help with stress and vice versa. Easing these symptoms will also have far-reaching health benefits.

If you have never been troubled with anxiety, stress or mental health issues, the appearance of symptoms of anxiety in menopause can be perplexing and confusing. If you have suffered with stress, anxiety or depression previously, menopause can trigger a worsening of symptoms. If menopause is recognised early on as an aggravating factor for these symptoms, taking appropriate action can reduce their severity and aid resolution.

Most of us know that it is important to talk about stress and anxiety, but this still remains a taboo subject in most situations. I strongly believe we need to bring this topic to the table because these symptoms are very common in menopause. It is important to talk about stress and anxiety because talking about it helps to defuse it (like defusing a bomb – more about that in Chapter 9).

Understanding the stress response and knowing how it can work against you in menopause can actually help you overcome many of the symptoms. It also helps those around you, especially your loved ones, to understand that anxiety adds another dimension to menopause and menopause adds another dimension to anxiety. Your mind and body are interlocking systems and cannot be separated in a binary way, so anxiety and stress also affect physical health. This can help explain many of the physical symptoms linked with anxiety.

I am going to start by describing some protective mechanisms, designed to combat and protect you from stress, that can become defective and destructive in today's modern world environment, and then I will show you how to biohack your stress response to make it work for you.

THE NATURE OF STRESS

Stress is a normal part of life. We are all built with the machinery to cope with sudden physical stress, but unrelenting stress can change the stress outcome from protective to harmful.

The limbic system (your emotional interpreter)

The stress response begins in the brain. Stressful stimuli are sensed and information is sent to the limbic system which controls emotional processing. The limbic system, interprets images and sounds (like a translator). When it perceives danger, it instantly sends warning signals to the hormone control centre in the brain (hypothalamus) and this cascades the fight or flight response.

In response to the limbic system stress signal, the hypothalamus sends signals to the autonomic nervous system; first the sympathetic and later the parasympathetic nervous systems.

Sympathetic nervous system (fight or flight)

The sympathetic nervous system functions like a fast-forward or accelerator pedal. It sends signals to the adrenal glands. These glands respond by pumping adrenaline into the bloodstream. This provides the body with a burst of energy so that it can respond to a threat. Other processes are subsequently triggered, including an increase in the heart rate and blood pressure, expanded air passages in the lungs and enlarged eye pupils, and extra blood is shunted to the muscles and brain. This is the 'fight or flight' response.

As the initial surge of adrenaline subsides, the second component of the stress response begins. This triggers release of the hormone cortisol from the adrenal glands. Cortisol keeps the body revved up and on high alert. The effects of cortisol include controlling the body's blood sugar levels, regulating metabolism, reducing inflammation, influencing memory and controlling salt and water balance and blood pressure.

Parasympathetic nervous system (rest and digest)

When the threat passes, fight or flight hormones fall. The parasympathetic nervous system then takes control and acts like a pause button or handbrake. It promotes the 'rest and digest' response that calms the body down after the danger has passed and it dampens the stress response.

MENOPAUSE NOW

Menopause symptoms can trigger stress and anxiety. Coupled with our enriched but increasingly busy lives, our modern world presents different types of external stress that our automatically programmed, protective stress responses are not prepared for. We are prepared for war and battle, interspersed with rest and recovery. Today stress is more likely to be relentless. This may be described as toxic or chronic stress and can result in accumulating 'stress debt' (recognised scientifically as 'allostatic load') and is harmful to the body in many ways.

Allostatic load

Allostasis refers to the complex processes that maintain the body's stress balance through the production of mediators such as adrenaline, cortisol and other chemical messengers. Allostatic load denotes wear and tear on the body, which can accumulate when an individual is exposed to repeated, relentless or chronic stress.

Although it is intuitive that chronic stress is likely to be harmful to physical health, stress is often dismissed as purely psychological. This is despite a large body of scientific literature relating to the negative health effects of allostatic load (toxic stress or stress debt).

Allostatic load was originally described in a landmark article published in the *Archives of Internal Medicine* journal in 1993. The authors set out to clarify ambiguities associated with the word 'stress'. They presented a new concept describing the relationship between chronic stress and the processes leading to physical disease, emphasising the hidden cost of chronic stress on the human body over time

If stressful stimuli are unrelenting, the human body can become unable to put the brakes on the stress response. Chronic low-level stress keeps the adrenal glands constantly revved up. If this imbalance in stress response is not resolved, the allostatic load accumulates and physical health problems associated with chronic stress can result.

Over time, repeated activation of the stress response can take its toll on the body. Brain changes may contribute to anxiety, depression and addiction. Research has shown that chronic stress contributes to high blood pressure and furring of arteries, as well as raising the risk of heart attacks and strokes. It can also contribute to weight gain and the build-up of fat tissue in the body. Additional negative effects on immune function and biorhythms can occur. It can even contribute to causing brittle bones.

> ## KEY FACT
>
> Chronic stress should not be considered as having only psychological effects, but as a genuine physical threat to health.

The stress response in menopause

We are all different and our individual susceptibilities – our personal 'stress signatures' – will contribute to our overall symptom burden during menopause. Our stress load will impact our physical health, risk of disease and indeed our menopause experience. Not everyone suffers from chronic stress, anxiety or mood issues in menopause – many women have none of these symptoms – but when they occur they can be very disruptive to health and well-being.

Menopause symptoms including insomnia, fatigue, palpitations, flushes and brain fog may relate to imbalances in the fight or flight response that can then trigger the psychological effects of anxiety. In this context, the fight or flight response becomes more harmful than helpful.

Biorhythms and the internal body clock can be disrupted by unbalanced stress and affect sleep quality and trigger fatigue, which can result in reduced physical activity and muscle aches and pains. Menopause is a stressful challenge on the body in itself, but external stress can lead to an increased burden of symptoms. Preventing, managing or reducing chronic stress can therefore have a beneficial impact on your whole menopause experience as well as your overall health.

MANAGING CHRONIC STRESS IN MENOPAUSE

In our modern world many women have not been able to build up the protective mechanisms to prevent modern-day chronic stress affecting their integrated health. Finding solutions can result in a rebalanced stress response and many long-term physical health benefits.

As early as possible, and certainly as you approach menopause, an important positive step is to find ways of 'rebalancing' and strengthening your stress response. The good news is that there are some relatively simple ways of doing this.

Firstly, physical activity, which produces a synchronised type of acute, healthy stress response, and a fall in stress hormones afterwards, assists with a healthy stress balance. How to build up physical activity sustainably in menopause is covered in Chapter 4. If you have not read this chapter yet, don't be put off by physical activity and be assured it is always possible to make time to do some. Any movement or activity is better than none. Micro-exercise is a great start – small, gradual changes can make all the difference. Exercise also has mindful-type properties, because when you are doing exercise or a focused physical activity, you are focusing your awareness on the present moment and this is a natural stress reliever.

Having a balanced diet might seem unrelated to stress, but it is linked and it is important. High-sugar food that can cause sugar crashes hours later can also cause brain fog and fatigue and these symptoms can pull mood downwards, worsen anxiety and put additional stress on the body. Sticking to unprocessed food and slow-release carbs will help with overall well-being and that is good for stress. Optimising micronutrients supports cellular energy metabolism and that is beneficial against stress. Food and nutrition are covered in greater detail in Chapters 5 and 8.

The next relatively simple action that can help with the overall stress response is re-establishing your circadian rhythm through good sleep patterns. I have included some detailed strategies to help with your sleep–wake cycle in Chapter 7, and sleep is a very important facet in physical stress management.

Anxiety tends to be made worse by pressure and deadlines. Being overcommitted and overburdened can result in you neglecting self-care. Pacing yourself by setting realistic short-term goals on a daily basis, and not overcommitting, will not only have a beneficial impact on your overall energy levels, but can be really helpful in averting anxiety and reducing the effects of stress. I will discuss pacing along with other fatigue management strategies in Chapter 11.

If you can be mindful of your commitments and utilise helpful lifestyle approaches before menopause, the stress component of symptoms will be lessened as you enter menopause. Some challenges and commitments are not possible to reduce, but many are, for example not taking on unnecessary additional voluntary roles or chores if you are already overburdened, not having excessively late nights out or overcommitting at work, and not bunching up social commitments. If you are able to adopt healthy lifestyle practices and a good life balance before menopause, this will almost certainly help with your overall health, productivity and well-being long-term, with no downside!

Mindfulness is a mind-management approach that helps enormously with stress management and this is covered in detail in Chapter 10. It is exceptionally helpful with balancing the physical stress response. It works by damping down the instinctive, emotional component of the stress response that is amplified (but ineffective) in chronic stress and augments the logical thought centre of the brain to trigger more appropriate actions. This can have far-reaching beneficial effects on your physical health.

The fact that these important lifestyle interventions to support stress management are covered in several other chapters – comprising my menopause toolkit – signifies the fact that stress is integrally linked with, and affected by, many body systems and networks and requires a multifaceted approach to management. If you have not yet read Chapters 4, 6, 7, 10 and 11, and if anxiety and stress are a major problem for you, then please read them now.

The majority of women in menopause do not need specialist management for anxiety or depression. If, however, anxiety symptoms and mood issues become severe and unrelenting this may suggest the development of an anxiety-related mood disorder. In this situation, it is important to be checked out by a doctor. Mood disorders, such as depression, can sometimes be flared up by menopause, especially if you have had a lot of previous major life events or traumas.

Prioritise stress-relieving pursuits

It is easy in a busy life to prioritise all the stressful tasks that you need to do, precluding the stress-relieving activities. You will, however, be better equipped to deal with the stressful and challenging matters in your life if you balance them with enjoyable activities and adequate relaxation.

Unrelenting standards and lack of self-compassion can often trick you into thinking you simply can't find the time to do the fun, stress-relieving activities that will help your well-being and reduce your stress. I always try to point out to my patients that if pushing their bodies to the extreme ends up making them ill, they will be of no use to their loved ones. Self-compassion and 'me time' are necessary pursuits in the achievement of stress relief, health and well-being. Fitting in these happy pursuits will be beneficial to all those around you.

In the following table I have listed some important strategies that you should try to include in your daily routine – they should not just be an occasional practice. These strategies aim to reduce the feeling of being under attack. A combination of these measures (rather than one used alone in isolation) can help with stress. You can then build on the techniques in a stepwise way to gain further benefit. These are my own recommendations from experience of supporting management of chronic stress and complex health issues using evidence-based practical approaches.

Simple techniques to reduce chronic stress

Technique	Step 1	Step 2
Take a breath of fresh air	Outdoor time whenever you can to blow away cobwebs, ideally on a daily basis	Regular outdoor walking, up to 30 minutes per day, will curb both physical and mental stress

Technique	Step 1	Step 2
Mindful breathing (basics of pranayama) – try to do this several times per day	Inhale, hold, exhale, hold. Try to do each for 3/4/5 seconds, repeat several times	Breathing ratios can be adjusted as you become familiar with the exercise with a ratio of 1:2:3
Exercise	Take a slowly, slowly approach to adding activity in to your life and then building it up	Ensure any programme is injury-proof
Ensure good nutrition to reduce brain fog and increase energy	Where possible, reduce high-sugar food and replace with natural high-fibre and complex carbs. Reduce wheat	Aim for a rainbow diet of unprocessed food
Be sleep-savvy	Try to establish a consistent sleep routine	Set a realistic sleep schedule and consolidate a regular bed and wake-up time
Ditch the tech. The average adult spends close to 11 hours looking at a screen per day and checks their phone every 10 minutes	Ensure some tech-free time each day	Go on a technology diet. Reduce your screen time by up to 2 hours per day if possible

Technique	Step 1	Step 2
Jettison the boom–bust approach	Try to be realistic about goals, commitments and deadlines (pace yourself) – this will make you more time-efficient and less under pressure	Keeping to a generally consistent (realistic) schedule will reduce stress debt
Me time	5 minutes doing something you enjoy once or twice a day	Take up a regular hobby of something you enjoy
Downtime	5 minutes stopping what you are doing to do nothing a couple of times per day	5–10 minutes of mindfulness practice (can use an app to help you), several times per day
Happy time	Anything that brings some laughter into your life, ideally on a daily basis	Regular time doing things that make you happy
Be mindful, don't catastrophise and introduce some self-compassion	When you have a negative thought, play a game of finding a positive spin on the thought	Learn about the practice of mindfulness
Address toxic relationships	Spend more time with people whose company you enjoy	Spend less time with the people who make you feel bad

Toxic relationships

Toxic relationships can be emotionally or physically damaging, and can relate to a partner, friend, colleague or family member. While a healthy relationship contributes to your self-esteem and emotional energy, a toxic relationship damages self-esteem, drains energy and increases stress and anxiety. In all your connections look for kindness, respect, compassion and an interest in your welfare. You should feel safe, comfortable, happy and secure without fear. In a toxic relationship you may feel insecure, dominated, belittled or controlled. This is not a safe place and my advice would be to distance yourself from this type of relationship wherever possible.

Spending time with people whose company you enjoy, doing activities that you enjoy, and laughing, are really good stress relievers. Anxiety and stress tend to be made worse by negative or toxic relationships so the less time spent in those situations, the better.

A quick recap

During menopause, stress can be triggered in a multitude of ways. You are born with the constitution to combat stress resulting from emergency situations that could threaten your survival. You were not built to automatically cope with the unrelenting stress that the modern world currently poses. This can create a significant challenge as you enter menopause and can influence your long-term health.

Confronting and overcoming modern-day chronic stress requires many overlapping techniques including regular physical activity, psychological approaches including relaxation and stress management techniques, self-compassion, pacing yourself, a good sleep–wake routine and good nutrition. These can all tend to be set at low priority during a busy menopause.

Understanding the important impact of the physical stress response on menopause and its symptoms should enable multiple modest changes to lower stress levels and reduce the overall burden of chronic stress with all its negative health effects. Eradicating stress debt can fight off many physical diseases and improve your long-term health.

CHAPTER 10

Menopause Mind

MENOPAUSE IS SUCH a busy time of life in today's world that your many different and varied roles can overload your brain – this can cause you to feel more stressed and anxious and it can make your brain foggy and forgetful. Simple mind-management approaches can ease stress, reduce anxiety and clear your mind.

For many years I have worked closely with colleagues who specialise in clinical psychology in relation to managing patients with various physical health issues. During this time, I have developed a good understanding of the importance of mind management – using psychological techniques – in the treatment of physical symptoms and hormone imbalance. These techniques add tremendous value when used together with other treatments, and improve outcomes for many conditions including menopausal symptoms. I can vouch for this myself as I have used informal mindfulness techniques to manage my own menopause in the context of a breast cancer diagnosis.

This chapter is based on my practical experience over many years. If you are suffering from lots of physical symptoms of menopause and/or have a lot of stress, reading this chapter should give you some useful understanding about why psychological techniques are helpful and how to implement some simple strategies to manage your symptoms.

I generally signpost my patients to psychological techniques that are likely to help with mood, motivation to make lifestyle changes, stress relief, brain fog, energy, well-being, hot flushes and sleep. I have learned a lot about these techniques over the years, but I am not a psychologist. This chapter is a whistle-stop guide to these techniques from a physician's perspective. For expert psychological advice please consult a qualified practitioner.

I sometimes observe a dismissive or defensive response when I mention psychological approaches such as mindfulness and cognitive behavioural therapy (CBT) to patients when I believe these may be helpful. The reasons for this are multiple. Stigma around the use of psychological approaches remains widespread, just like there is still stigma around mental health in general. When symptoms are unexplained or difficult to resolve and a doctor asks you to consider psychological approaches, there can be a frustration that the doctor is suggesting it's 'all in your mind' when you know it is not. You may be cynical about the approaches and have doubts about their usefulness, but they do add value. Implementing mind-management techniques is not an easy practice but, once mastered, can be an extremely useful tool in managing symptoms of menopause.

WHAT EXACTLY IS MINDFULNESS?

Mindfulness describes the awareness that arises from being voluntarily fully present in our current surroundings, being non-judgemental about where we are and what we're doing, and not overly reactive to or overwhelmed by what's going on around us. Although mindfulness originated in Buddhism, modern mindfulness approaches are generally secular.

There is good evidence that mindfulness-based techniques help with many aspects of quality of life. Mindfulness-based stress reduction (MBSR) techniques have also been shown to help with hot flushes in menopause.

THE SEVEN PILLARS OF MINDFULNESS

1. Non-judgement: just observing, witnessing.
2. Patience: allowing things to unfold in their own time.
3. Beginner's mind: observing with a fresh pair of eyes.
4. Trust: trust yourself, your feelings, your own intuition and wisdom.
5. Non-striving: non-doing, less is more.
6. Acceptance: come to terms with how things are right now.
7. Letting go: don't cling on to thoughts, feelings and judgements.

(Adapted from: Kabat-Zinn, J. (2004), *Full Catastrophe Living: How to cope with stress, pain and illness using mindfulness meditation.*)

The father of MBSR is considered by some to be Jon Kabat-Zinn, Emeritus Professor of Medicine at the University of Massachusetts Medical School, who brought this practice into the mainstream after an epiphany moment almost 40 years ago.

MBSR is a cognitive approach in which you are taught to notice a symptom in a non-judgemental way. This allows you to be aware of a symptom and any associated negative thought that accompanies it. This noticing and awareness can help reduce the tendency to react to these thoughts. It allows you to objectively view the thoughts as just thoughts and separate them from current reality. You may be able to do this simply by practising it yourself. If not, and you want to learn, you can do a MBSR course as they are now quite widely available.

An example of a situation that can be influenced by your stress response is you going to an important function (a party or work do). You are not sure what to wear and don't know a lot of the people going. If your stress response is healthy then you can rein in negative thoughts and keep perspective. You will be your true self, meet some new people and enjoy the event.

Now consider if your stress response is overloaded – you are literally 'stressed out'. Your mind may have recurring thoughts of, 'My outfit is all wrong', 'I have no idea what to say to people, they will think I am dull' or 'What if I have a massive sweat or flush?' This takes you away from the reality of the here and now and you may be less likely to feel chatty and friendly and more likely to have the dreaded sweating attack because you are so stressed. You can become so preoccupied with *thinking* about the worst-case scenario that your thoughts can make it more likely to happen.

Noticing your thoughts

If you find yourself in that dreaded emotionally stressful situation you can counteract it using a technique called 'defusion'. When a repeated thought response to a situation is 'I can't cope' it can make the situation feel more stressful. If this thought is overridden and separated from the situation with the thought 'I am thinking I can't cope', this can create some psychological space from the initial unhelpful thought. If a further override step is added – 'I am noticing the thought that I can't cope' – this highlights to the conscious mind that the thought is a thought and not reality, and can reduce the negative impact of the experience and help with your stress levels.

DEFUSION: A NOTICING EXERCISE

1. Say 'I can't cope' repeatedly for one minute.
2. Then say 'I am thinking I can't cope' repeatedly for one minute.

> 3. Then say 'I am noticing I am thinking I can't cope'
>   repeatedly for one minute.

Notice how you feel when you repeat each version. It is likely that you will feel much less bad with the third version than the first.

The term for the process of counteracting negative thoughts is known as 'nonreactive awareness' to an experience. Your emotional mind constantly judges. Nonreactive awareness or 'noticing' allows your logical mind to notice what your emotional mind is doing, and this reduces the impact of that judgement on how you feel and your stress response.

To give you another example, a woman may react to a hot flush with feelings of impending doom and catastrophe:

- 'It is horrible – it seems never-ending and is destroying my sleep.'
- 'It is always happening at the worst possible times during the day; other people must notice and must be judging me.'
- 'I am covered in sweat, they will think I am so weird with perspiration running down my cheeks.'
- 'I am a freak, no one could possibly understand this.'
- 'It's like a prison sentence.'

The mindfulness-based approach would put the brakes on those negative thought processes and judgements. Defusion techniques can be used to allow you to label the hot flush just as a hot flush, something temporary, and while it may be uncomfortable, it will go away. This approach puts a stop to paying symptoms any more attention than they deserve. Adding compassionate logical thoughts can also help, such as, 'Other people will not notice what

I am noticing, this is actually a normal occurrence in menopause and many other women are going through this too and will understand,' which is all true.

Creating pausitivity

The positive change in your perception of the experience, what is sometimes called 'pausitivity', actually reduces the stress component of the whole situation and this can alter the outcome in a positive way. This is the case in many health settings. It can be used for many other distressing symptoms of menopause, including fatigue, brain fog, insomnia, palpitations and low mood.

Slow and steady wins the race

If menopause symptoms start to slow you down, you may pursue boom-and-bust approaches to daily tasks to try to get as much done as possible. A common example is housework – trying to do it all at once and ending up exhausted rather than tackling one room or one floor at a time over a few days – or doing all the washing and ironing at once rather than spacing it out. You may use similar approaches to work and social activities. This mindset can actually result in you getting less done because it can produce a worn-out and weary version of yourself. Things can then take longer or end up unfinished. Try to remember that slow and steady is more efficient, productive and sustainable.

Tempering your expectations and being more realistic about what you can reliably achieve can make a seismic difference to your energy balance. In particular, this can allow you to have a steady level day to day, rather than a roller-coaster activity ride. You will get more done that way. This certainly requires prioritising activity and sometimes not committing to certain things, which can feel counter-intuitive. Overriding these emotive instincts with active logical thought insertion is not an automatic process and requires active reflection and circumspection. This is where mindfulness becomes a winning ticket. Cognitive and mindfulness approaches can be very helpful in rationalising busy thought processes.

Mindfulness-based thinking approaches are not a solution for all symptoms, life events and illnesses – they were never meant to be the answer to all of life's complexities – but better outcomes have been observed for many conditions with mindfulness techniques. They can help people get on with their lives, with enriched enjoyment, alongside symptoms. MBSR techniques and CBT (see page 133) have been shown to improve hot flushes, stress and other symptoms in menopause.

Being fully in the present moment, and limiting how much time you invest in paying attention to your emotional thoughts and symptoms, you will be much better able to notice the reality of the here and now and also choose your behavioural response to symptoms carefully.

Although the full extent of mindfulness and CBT techniques require time and support with a supervised treatment course, implementing some of the simple mindfulness strategies that I have described can be self-taught and there are also online mindfulness applications and programmes that can help you learn and build on the basic skills yourself. Informal mindfulness practices do not require formal supervision or training and don't take up additional time as they simply involve paying conscious and voluntary attention to what you are *already* doing.

EVERYDAY MINDFULNESS

Below are some examples of informal mindfulness techniques that are easy to build into your daily life, enrich it and reduce stress. You can use these like a prescription and try to build some of them into your daily routine, ideally several times per day for short periods. It might seem strange at first, but after a while you will see how these simple techniques can distract your emotional centre from judging and bring your logical mind into the driving seat. Some of these practices are also used in more formal mindfulness practices, but if you can discipline yourself to practise them independently on a daily basis they will be greatly beneficial.

Self-compassion

Notice when you're being harsh and judgemental with yourself and guide your thoughts towards self-compassion. This is so important in menopause and for women in general. It is probably the most important mindfulness practice that you can use to improve your well-being.

Walking outside

(My favourite!) Walk outside even for 10 minutes, but for as long as you are able to commit. Don't take your ear-pods! Listen to nature: the birds singing, dogs barking, wind howling, fallen leaves rustling. Notice the cold air on your cheeks, the rain drops or the sun's heat on your skin. Listen to all the other 'here-and-now' events happening: workmen with machinery, vehicles driving past, planes flying above, sirens sounding. Notice what you see: houses up for sale, new buildings being constructed, people walking by chatting, and many other things I have not mentioned.

Eating meditation

Focus mindfully on a piece of food as you fully experience the smell, texture, taste and other sensations of the food as you eat it very slowly. This is good to do anyway, every day, because eating slowly is good for digestion and appetite control.

Showering

Feel the sensations and warmth of the water. Listen to the sound of the spray of the water around you. Notice your thoughts and feelings as you take in the entire experience of the shower.

Driving

Pay attention to what you see, the feel of the steering wheel in your hands and what you're hearing around you. Relax your shoulders and notice what you're feeling and experiencing as you mindfully drive.

Breathing

Your breath is always with you and you don't need a formal practice to benefit from breath awareness. Pausing at any time throughout your day to connect to your breath and notice yourself inhaling and exhaling is an important part of informal as well as formal mindfulness practice. (See Chapter 7 for more on this.)

Body scanning

Slowly and intentionally scan your body with your mind from the top of your head to the tips of your toes, noticing any symptoms without judging them.

COMBATING UNHELPFUL THOUGHTS

Something that people often fail to realise is that if we are continually distracted by multiple thoughts and our minds are too busy and full, we tend not to be mindful. Our default is to make instinctive and negative judgements much of the time and this can give rise to emotional thoughts running away with us. At worst, this can result in a tendency to 'catastrophise'; that is to perceive any number of situations as considerably worse than they actually are.

Your emotion thought control centre in the brain is called the limbic system (see also page 120). It is a complex network that underpins behaviour, mood and memory. It retrieves information from your senses about what is happening around you in the current moment and triggers the fight or flight response when there is danger. If your limbic system decides to create an infinite loop of negative or unhelpful thoughts that are not actually linked with your current reality, this can switch on the stress response even though there is, in reality, no acute threat. The limbic system can therefore 'bypass' the sight and sound senses, because it is anticipating danger and generates a recurring loop of stress thoughts. This is a protective mechanism gone wrong and is a relatively common scenario in today's world in many situations, not just menopause.

Often your instinctive reactions to your menopause symptoms come from the emotional thought centre in your brain. It is trying to help but it does not always gauge the situation correctly in our modern world and can influence you to react in the wrong way by creating unhelpful thoughts. Mind-management techniques, generated by your logical mind, are a way of reining in your over-committed emotional thought centre, which amplifies your stress response, overriding these thoughts and promoting more appropriate actions that will deactivate the stress response when it is not needed. You can therefore actually change your responses in a positive way and ultimately improve your symptoms.

Taming the hormonsters

If your emotional thought centre is allowed to run your stress response to virtual (theoretical) threats of stress, many menopausal symptoms can run wild. If your emotional thought centre is trained to respond appropriately to current reality, by being kept in check by your logical thought centre, many symptoms related to stress will reduce or disappear.

Let's say you are super-busy and you start to forget silly things, like the name of someone you have known for ages, or you make mistakes like putting your house keys in the fridge. There are lots of simple mistakes we all make when we are overstretched and stressed. If your emotional thought centre is left unchecked, you could easily develop a thought loop that tells you that you are getting dementia. These recurring thoughts will make you feel sad, low and more anxious, even panicked. They may affect your sleep and you will feel more tired and will be more likely to be forgetful and have reduced concentration and focus, so the cycle will perpetuate itself.

If, with the same symptoms, your logical mind reminds you that you are overstretched and that is why you are being forgetful, you will not give the simple mistakes unnecessary attention and you will rightly feel more compassionate towards yourself. Then you will be more likely to make some lifestyle changes to take the pressure off, such as trying to overcommit less and allowing yourself some 'me time'. This will reduce your forgetfulness, help your sleep and improve fatigue.

Simply raising logical awareness and thinking 'mindfully' is a powerful tool to reduce stress and lessen symptoms. Whenever I get a negative or self-loathing thought I try very hard to think of a logical balanced argument and it almost always reduces my stress, which makes me more productive, less tired and more tolerant. Of course, there will always be times when doing that can be difficult, but if counterbalancing your emotional mind with your logical mind is the only mindful-based strategy you utilise, it will still be transforming.

In the following table I have outlined some more examples of emotional thought loops that can make symptoms worse and a logical mind response that can counteract them. When you notice unhelpful thoughts, you can introduce them to logical thoughts that will be more helpful and hopefully override the instinctive unhelpful ones. You may recognise some of the scenarios; if so, try to focus on the logical response more that the emotional context.

A quick recap

Spending too much time thinking negative or random thoughts can be draining. It can also make you more likely to experience stress, anxiety, foggy brain and low mood. Your emotional mind centre needs to be balanced by your logical mind activity.

How to balance your emotional thought centre with your logical mind centre

Symptom	Instinctive unhelpful thought	Use defusion and then replace with logical counter-thought	Even better thoughts	Do not think this way and do not catastrophise
Insomnia	I can't sleep. It's hopeless, I can't function without sleep	When I am in bed I am resting, even though I am not asleep all through the night. I will eventually get to sleep. I have the tools to get started on improving my sleep	I am going to overhaul my sleep rituals, have no screen time for 2 hours before bed and I will practise mindful breathing techniques when needed	I must sleep during the day whenever I can to make up for lack of sleep at night
Fatigue	I am exhausted – it is always the same. I need to go back to bed today. This must be due to something really serious	Sleep is not the answer to my exhaustion. If I sleep a lot I don't feel better. Fatigue is caused by many different factors and I need to work on all of them. This will take time	I am going to keep a diary and make small changes, avoid boom–bust activity, apply more self-care and be realistic with goals	I am staying in bed; my body is telling me to

Symptom	Instinctive unhelpful thought	Use defusion and then replace with logical counter-thought	Even better thoughts	Do not think this way and do not catastrophise
Weight gain	I have eaten virtually nothing for the last week and I have hardly lost any weight. I don't have time to focus on healthy eating – ready meals are quicker. I must have a problem that stops me losing weight	My weight has gone on over a few years so I need to pace myself with weight loss. Small changes will be more effective	Ready meals are more expensive and less nutritious. I can try making some easy, healthy dishes that don't take too much time	I can't cook and don't have time to shop
Stress	I have too much to do; I cannot cope	I need some downtime each day or I will get burned out and I won't get as much done. I am going to write a list of priorities. I will reach out to family and friends for support	I will be more efficient if I don't stress and take things in my stride. Asking for help is a good idea	I will never get everything done, it's hopeless

143

Symptom	Instinctive unhelpful thought	Use defusion and then replace with logical counter-thought	Even better thoughts	Do not think this way and do not catastrophise
Anxiety	My anxiety is uncontrollable – my whole body is shaking, I cannot breathe, I feel like I am suffocating	It is likely that I am having a panic attack. I need to stop what I am doing and focus on my breathing and try to eradicate the negative thoughts	I will look at triggers. I am going to limit caffeine and alcohol. I am going to use relaxation techniques and increase my exercise. I will talk to my doctor about having formal cognitive therapy	There is something seriously wrong, perhaps a heart attack

Practising mindfulness exercises can help you direct your attention away from emotional negative thinking and activate logical thoughts. This will reduce stress-related symptoms and enable you to engage positively with the world around you.

Acceptance and self-compassion are not attitudes that are easily or spontaneously adopted in menopause, particularly when you are stressed and have just behaved irrationally, irritably or out of character. You are more likely to have feelings of self-loathing, which will make you feel worse. If you understand the biology underpinning your symptoms, you will be more likely to adopt some self-care and choose to implement mind-management techniques, such as mindfulness, to help you utilise your logical mind centre to balance your thoughts and manage these situations.

CHAPTER 11

Overcoming Fatigue

TIRED ALL THE time? Lost that sparkle? Fatigue can hold its own in the league table of menopausal symptoms. There are very few women who consult with me about menopause who say fatigue is not an issue for them. Medical causes can play a role, but for most of us this symptom has many diverse and varied contributory causes.

There are many modern-world factors that are making fatigue a greater problem for women today compared to a generation ago. It is a complex symptom with very tangled roots and needs a multifaceted and holistic approach, as well as perseverance, to overcome. Conquering fatigue in menopause has tremendous benefits to quality of life.

The reason fatigue can be so perplexing is that every system in the human body makes a contribution to energy. If one single system fails, for example you develop liver or kidney failure, fatigue is clearly explained by blood tests and scans, and the treatment path is usually obvious. If, as is the case in menopause, there is imbalance affecting several body systems, but no single system or zone has actually failed, there may be no blood test or scan that will explain it.

MENOPAUSE NOW

Fatigue is worse for many women today because they are juggling menopause with so many more commitments – they are part of a 'sandwich' generation, with time needed to support elderly parents, dependent kids, challenging work and voluntary roles. Overcommitment can result in chronic stress and seemingly less time for much-needed exercise. Technology in the bedroom disrupts sleep. Poor-quality food, that is labelled to look healthy can result in deficiencies of essential micronutrients. These factors can all contribute to menopause fatigue.

CASE HISTORY: COLETTE

Colette came to see me in my clinic due to severe menopausal symptoms. She was absolutely exhausted. Her symptoms had worsened over one year. She was 48 and having heavy periods. Her insomnia led her to try to get extra sleep at different times, so she was napping a lot in the daytime. She had no energy to cook food from scratch so was living on ready meals. She had stopped her exercise programme because of her fatigue and her weight was increasing.

Winter arrived and Colette fell ill with the flu and was wiped out for much longer than anyone else she knew who had the same bug. Colette had already been underperforming at work due to brain fog and needed quite a lot of time off work during the flu infection. She ended up in a stressful disciplinary work situation. She couldn't afford not to work but knew she was not able to do her job properly. Her mood crashed and she was worried that she would lose her job. Colette went to see her doctor, who told her that there was nothing wrong with her. He said that her symptoms were not related to menopause because she was still having periods. She was offered an antidepressant. She came to see me in utter desperation. She didn't believe that her severe fatigue and other physical symptoms were all down to depression, although by the time she saw me, after a year of terrible quality of life, she was starting to feel depressed.

This management of Colette is wrong on many levels. When menopause symptoms begin, they will often be dismissed by healthcare professionals or, worse still, incorrectly diagnosed as something else, like depression. This problem comes from our healthcare culture, which only accepts clear-cut, tangible diseases that show up on blood tests and scans. If you feel unwell and don't have a blood test or scan to show for it you may well be left in the wilderness.

Colette had no idea what her menopausal symptoms were or how to deal with them when they started. She was in fact told that it was not menopause. She believed that sleeping more was the answer to her insomnia and fatigue. She believed that the ready meals would be giving her all the nutrients she needed; after all, the packaging looked healthy and she was gaining weight, not losing it. As she felt ill she thought it best to stop exercise and activity. Her work problems triggered stress and mood issues, which created a vicious cycle. Being told by her GP that there was nothing wrong with her led her to feel hopeless.

I explained to Colette that her symptoms were likely to be significantly related to menopause, even though she was still having periods, but that things had got out of control for several reasons. Her coping strategies were not fit for purpose. She needed to create a sleep routine, and she needed to try to move around more to loosen up her aching muscles. She was eating food that was high in calories and low in nutrients but the labelling was deceptive and led Colette to believe that her diet was balanced. In fact, she was likely to be deficient in some energy-boosting micronutrients, including iron because of her heavy periods and possibly B vitamins, both of which can worsen brain fog in menopause. I explained that as it was winter Colette was likely to be vitamin D deficient and this could be contributing to her muscle aches and low immunity. I explained that deficiency in vitamin D and other micronutrients such as zinc and B vitamins may have contributed to her poor recovery from the flu and worsening symptoms of fatigue and I explained that everyone feels more fatigued after an infection, so that in itself was also contributing to her symptom burden. Having all these problems on top of menopause culminated in severe symptoms.

Colette immediately felt quite liberated when she understood what was going on. It all made sense to her. Lots of small factors had added together and produced a hugely amplified negative effect on her well-being. She approached her symptoms one by one and accepted that the fatigue would not miraculously improve immediately with each action but gradual, incremental benefits would become evident in time. Colette had mild anaemia, a borderline low B12, folate and zinc, and very low vitamin D. (Her GP blood test had found the mild anaemia but this was said to be 'normal' because her periods were heavy.) Colette modified her diet and was able to take a non-prescription vitamin and mineral supplement. Her brain fog lifted quickly and her energy gradually improved. She was able to return to work, performing better. She set out to work on her sleep, activity and stress management. She felt empowered and wanted to delay a decision to take hormone therapy but she was aware that this was an option depending on her progress.

Colette is a good example that fatigue is frequently complex and multifactorial and addressing one single important issue may not restore health and well-being because other contributory factors may not have been identified and rectified. This is a perfect example of my 'house of menopause' metaphor (see pages 30–1).

GETTING TO THE ROOT CAUSE OF FATIGUE

Fatigue is frequently not straightforward to unravel. Family doctors have very tight time constraints in consultations, making it extremely challenging for them to identify the root causes. As a consequence, symptoms of unexplained fatigue are frequently given a diagnostic label of 'tired all the time' by doctors. I believe this is an unhelpful label and it does not rectify the problem.

So-called 'red flag' features that doctors will investigate are generally looking for a single unifying diagnosis that will not pick up complex causes or identify the multifaceted management needed for someone like Colette described above.

To help you understand just how complex the underlying causes of fatigue can be, I have included a table below explaining several different 'energy zones', which are invisible and which can all contribute to an end result of a seemingly simple symptom of fatigue. You will see that many are interchangeable. Almost all of these are in your power to change if you understand what changes to make – and these are often very simple things. I have therefore explained what actions might make your symptoms worse and those that will improve them.

Some energy-loss zones causing fatigue in menopause

Energy zone	Made worse by	Made better by
Infections (immune system)	Micronutrient deficiencies, chronic stress, lack of sleep	A to Z supplement, sleep routine, stress management
Stress response and anxiety	Worry, major life events, depression, brain fog, sweats, overcommitted	Relaxation, exercise, mindfulness, self-compassion, pacing
Diet and nutrition	Processed foods, extreme low- or high-carb diets, or other restrictive diets. Dietary intolerances, IBS, bowel disorders	Cooking from scratch, healthy balance, limiting foods that worsen symptoms (avoid/limit packets, jars and ready meals)
Sleep	More than nine or fewer than six hours per night and excessive daytime sleep	Regular night sleep routine, avoid blue light screens and use relaxation techniques before bed
Activity level	Too sedentary, frequent daytime naps, bed days, overexertion	Paced regular daily activity, preferably outdoors

Energy zone	Made worse by	Made better by
Organisation	Deadlines, boom-and-bust approach	Activity pacing, planning, interspersing activity with rest, don't bunch up high-stress events close together
Genetic	If you have had fatigue for your whole life	Combination of healthy lifestyle approaches, can try supplements such as CoQ10. *Seek medical help*
Menopause mind	Unrelenting standards, boom-and-bust approach, anxiety, disorganisation	Acceptance, planning, mindfulness, interspersing activity with rest, supplements to help brain fog such as zinc and B vitamins
Chronic pain	Many pain drugs	Gradually increasing activity, CBT and lifestyle approaches
Mood	Depression, boredom, lack of acceptance	Exercise, stress management, sunlight exposure, some supplements such as St John's wort (not if on prescription medication)

Energy zone	Made worse by	Made better by
Work and education	Toxic work stress, unsupportive employer, deadlines	Supportive employer, deadline extensions, compassionate working environment
Hormone imbalance	Fluctuating perimenopause and other hormone issues such as thyroid problems	Smoothing the hormone levels with treatment adjustments, phytoestrogens or HRT. *Seek medical help*
Drugs	Too many prescriptions or supplements that can interact	Rationalise the treatments, revert to lifestyle measures where possible. *Seek medical help*
Major life events	Stress, trauma	CBT/bereavement counselling/EMDR therapy. *Seek medical help*
Weight	Too high or too low	Steady, gradual, objective approach to weight management. *Seek medical help*
Coexisting health issues	Anaemia, migraine, fibromyalgia, arthritis, hypothyroidism, diabetes, heart problems	*Seek medical help and support*

Energy zone	Made worse by	Made better by
Hydration level	Not drinking enough fluids, dehydration	Ensure you drink no less than 1.2 litres and up to 3 litres of fluid per day depending on your exercise level, sweating level and weather temperature

When to ask for help from your doctor

It is difficult to give specific guidance here because there are an infinite number of potential causes of fatigue. If you feel very unwell you should seek help from your doctor. In particular, if you have implemented logical lifestyle approaches and symptoms of fatigue continue to be severe or if you have new progressive symptoms, such as unexplained weight loss or weight gain, severe headaches that you cannot link with menopause or lifestyle issues, then you should ask your GP for help. This help should involve, at the least, a clinical assessment and blood tests to look for additional, potential treatable causes of your symptoms.

Doctors have good clinical assessment skills to assess for sinister causes, so those will generally be identified quite swiftly by a doctor. When these tests are normal you can be reassured that there is no sinister or progressive disease and it is likely that a combination of dovetailed approaches, outlined below, will help relieve your fatigue going forward.

HOW TO RELIEVE FATIGUE

There are many factors within your control that you can change to improve fatigue-related symptoms, and we have covered many of these in the previous chapters. Stress, sleep dysfunction, poor diet, low nutrient levels, physical weakness, too much alcohol, pain and low mood can all contribute to, worsen or directly cause symptoms of fatigue. The good news is that the more factors linked to fatigue you can address, the more robust your energy and well-being infrastructure will become, and improvements in symptoms of fatigue and well-being are likely to follow.

We have already seen the importance of activity management, nutrition and sleep quality for supporting a healthy menopause. In addition to these factors, addressing stress management and utilising mindfulness techniques are also major players in successful fatigue management and these are discussed in detail in Chapters 9 and 10. If, therefore, you can successfully implement the recommendations from my other toolkit chapters, you will be well on your way to improving your overall energy and vitality.

Pace yourself

Another energy loss zone in menopause relates to simply overdoing things on an ongoing basis. This can inadvertently be quite a depleting pursuit. It is a bit like going to the bank and withdrawing enough money to last you for a week and then spending it in one day. Then you go back to the bank and say you need more to get you through. The bank, however, not only refuses to give you more, but charges interest on what has been borrowed. This is a metaphor for your energy! In menopause, if you expend too much energy in one go, you have effectively borrowed it and then have to pay back the excess, so you are incapacitated for a while until you have saved up some more energy. The way to prevent these energy fluctuations, which can be very debilitating, is to use a strategy called 'pacing'.

If you need to get something done it is instinctive to push yourself as hard as possible to complete the task because you can tell yourself that if you don't do it, you may let people down. But the reality is that no one is indispensable and most things can wait. Prioritising your commitments is likely to improve your productivity. You will be able to do more for yourself and others if you look after yourself. Pacing yourself, by setting realistic short-term goals on a daily basis and not overcommitting, will have a beneficial impact on your overall energy levels, which will remain more steady and reduce your fatigue. It can also be really helpful in averting anxiety and reducing the effects of stress. Being mindful that if you pace yourself you are less likely to end up exhausted and unproductive will allow you to rethink your commitments and create a more realistic schedule that includes self-care.

Micromanagement of multiple seemingly small contributors to low energy can be incredibly effective at unscrambling fatigue and can translate into a robust gradual improvement in well-being. If you can focus on conserving even tiny fractions of energy in different zones of your body, they will gradually and steadily all add up to a significant gain in well-being and vitality.

Manage symptom setbacks

If you embrace all the lifestyle approaches needed to improve your symptoms of tiredness and start to see your mojo returning, but then have a setback such as a chest infection or the flu, this can feel like you are back to square one. That is not the case. Improvements in fatigue are almost never linear, and there can be blips along the way. Improvement will follow a wavy line, and a downward dip with a setback is just that. It will take an upturn once the hurdle is passed.

In the following table I have summarised the main trigger factors for fatigue that you can address yourself to improve your overall energy and well-being. The more factors you can address, the greater the positive impact will be on your symptoms.

Factors at play in menopause fatigue and self-management

Fatigue trigger factor	Management approach
Too much activity, overcommitted and unrelenting standards	Pacing, CBT, mindfulness approaches, activity management
Too much rest	Activity management, build up activity
Poor dietary choices	Simplify diet, exclude processed food especially sugar
Nutritional factors	Consider an A to Z supplement
Insomnia and sleep issues	Sleep hygiene, cognitive techniques, mindfulness approaches
Too much alcohol	It is an unhelpful coping strategy, as is smoking – cut back or stop
Stress	Mindfulness-based stress management
Chronic aches and pains	CBT, graded activity, mindfulness approaches
Low mood	CBT, mindfulness approaches, consider fish oils and vitamin D
Negative thinking	CBT, mindfulness approaches
Other medical problems not optimised	*Seek medical help*
Full house of menopause symptoms despite lifestyle interventions	Hormone therapy or non-hormone alternatives should be considered

A quick recap

Fatigue is a troublesome symptom that is very common during menopause. It has a wide range of driving factors. Using a combination of systematic and prescriptive approaches can make a sizeable impact on symptoms of fatigue, even if one measure used alone doesn't seem to help. Understanding the strategies that work for fatigue is important because these can sometimes be counter-intuitive; for example many people with fatigue sleep too much! None of us are perfect and there will always be some strategies you find easier than others to implement, but if you are aware about what will help, you will automatically make some changes for the better and that will gradually translate into improved well-being, vitality and hopefully getting your mojo back.

CHAPTER 12

Bone Health

PEAK BONE STRENGTH is achieved around your mid- to late twenties. After that, bone strength falls with age (see illustration below). As we are living longer than any generation before us, keeping your bones strong as you get older is more important than ever. Broken bones can be serious and can be a consequence of brittle bones (also known as osteoporosis). The risk of brittle bones is affected by many genetic and health factors, including:

- smoking
- drinking too much alcohol
- not enough physical activity
- chronic stress
- inadequate dietary calcium
- vitamin D deficiency
- having an early menopause
- living a long life into old age

Understanding your individual risk can therefore help you recognise what you can do for yourself to keep your bones strong in your postmenopause years. Until a broken bone occurs there are typically no symptoms associated with brittle bones.

BONE LOSS DUE TO MENOPAUSE

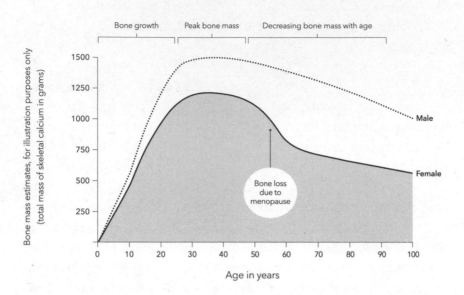

FACTORS INFLUENCING BONE STRENGTH

Many lifestyle factors can affect bone health and bone strength after menopause. If you feel that you have a lot of risk factors for bone thinning you should consider discussing this with your doctor.

KEY FACT

One of the most important contributors to bone health throughout life is a balanced diet. Ensuring that you obtain all the nutrients required for healthy bones throughout life is crucial.

Calcium and vitamin D

Two micronutrients that are particularly important for bone health throughout life are calcium and vitamin D.

Calcium

Calcium is an essential mineral and is extremely important in building and maintaining bone strength throughout your life. Without enough calcium in your diet, you may be at increased risk of osteoporosis.

Dairy products are a good source of calcium. Dairy also contains other important nutrients for bone health, such as phosphorus, magnesium and protein. Fortified non-dairy milk also contains vitamin D, but cow's milk does not.

In recent decades, there has been a noteworthy change in dietary patterns. Dairy has received some bad press. Some studies have indicated that dairy may protect against cancer, while others suggest that dairy may increase cancer risk. Dairy and lactose intolerance is being more frequently diagnosed.

Depending on what people read about dairy, many more people are choosing dairy-free diets because they perceive they will achieve beneficial health effects. Vegan diets are also increasing in popularity for a number of reasons.

Excluding dairy from your diet does not mean that you will not be able to obtain enough calcium for healthy bones. Many non-dairy milk alternatives are fortified with calcium and vitamin D. If, however, you are not savvy and are not checking the amount of calcium you are consuming (whether you are dairy-free or just don't eat much dairy) you may be inadvertently leaving your bones short on calcium and that can silently result in bone thinning, undetected right up to the point you get an unexpected bone fracture years or decades later.

It is recommended that after menopause women require 1200mg calcium per day. There is a fantastic food fact sheet produced by the Association of UK Dietitians that shows you how much calcium is in common food groups. You can access it here: https://www.bda.uk.com/resource/calcium.html

This shows good dairy and non-dairy sources of calcium. If you have a dairy-free or vegan diet you must ensure you are getting enough calcium. It should not be necessary for most women in menopause to take extra calcium supplements, with the exception of people who cannot achieve the 1200mg through their diet. It should also be noted that dietary calcium intake in excess of this amount can have negative effects, including kidney stones. Higher amounts of dietary calcium have no additional benefit on bone health.

Vitamin D

Vitamin D is a very important micronutrient for bone health because it helps your intestines absorb calcium from the food you eat. In its activated form, after changes are made to it in the liver and kidneys, more bone-strengthening effects occur. It is therefore very important in both the prevention and treatment of osteoporosis. Getting enough vitamin D is an important part of making sure your bones are dense and strong. Vitamin D is actually a hormone and seems to have effects in the body beyond bone health. For example, it has been shown to have important immune system effects. The role of the liver and kidneys in the bone-strengthening actions of activated vitamin D means that people with liver and kidney problems can be more at risk of bone problems and osteoporosis.

Vitamin D is sometimes called the 'sunshine vitamin' because it is made in the skin when it is exposed to direct sunlight or, in particular, ultraviolet-B radiation (UVB). The body can also obtain vitamin D through dietary sources, where it is found mainly in oily fish, such as mackerel, tuna and salmon, egg yolk and fortified foods such as breakfast cereals.

In the UK, and at similar latitudes, summer midday sunlight contains enough UVB light for vitamin D synthesis, while the weaker sunlight of winter provides a negligible amount of vitamin D synthesis. Therefore, vitamin D status declines throughout the winter. To remain sufficient in vitamin D all year round, a relatively high circulating level of vitamin D must be achieved by the end of the summer through sun exposure.

Melanin pigment in your skin absorbs ultraviolet radiation (UVR) and protects underlying skin from damage caused by UVR. It also reduces the UVR available for vitamin D synthesis in the skin. If you have darker or olive skin, and do not tend to burn easily, you can be more susceptible to vitamin D deficiency, while if you have pale skin that has a tendency to burn, you will achieve sufficient levels of vitamin D with lower sun exposure, but you may be more likely to need to use sunscreen to prevent sunburn damage.

Vitamin D deficiency can become a problem if you have inadequate sun exposure during the summer due to adverse weather, staying mostly indoors, due to skin type or through the use of sunscreen, because sunscreen prevents vitamin D absorption and it's hard to balance skin protection with getting enough vitamin D. Without supplementation, there is generally not enough vitamin D obtained from food sources in modern diets to make up for inadequate sunlight exposure.

UK government advice on vitamin D supplementation from the Department of Health changed in 2016 after the acknowledgement that most people in the UK would not be able to achieve adequate vitamin D levels for optimal health in the winter months. Between late March/early April and September, the majority of adults will probably obtain sufficient vitamin D from sunlight when they are outdoors, alongside foods that naturally contain or are fortified with vitamin D. As such, they might choose not to take a vitamin D supplement during these months.

Government recommendations state that from October to March everyone over the age of five years will need to rely on dietary sources of vitamin D. Since vitamin D is found only in a small number of foods, it might be difficult to get enough from foods that naturally contain vitamin D and/or fortified foods alone. The guidance therefore suggests that everyone should consider taking a daily supplement containing 10mcg of vitamin D. This guidance does not single out women in menopause for special recommendations. However, it does state that for individuals with low sunlight exposure all year round, an all-year-round vitamin D supplement should be considered. In other Western countries, vitamin D is fortified in many dairy products. In the UK, dairy is not generally fortified with vitamin D as standard, but non-dairy alternatives are.

Other vitamins and minerals

There has been interest in the role of several other vitamins and minerals on bone health, but no clear-cut role in osteoporosis prevention or treatment after menopause has been found. Eating a balanced diet and paying attention to all the micronutrients discussed in Chapter 5 should be safe and beneficial. Interest in the roles of vitamin K, magnesium and other nutrients on bone health continues, but it's still not clear if supplementing them is beneficial in menopause.

One nutrient that needs caution is vitamin A. Some research has suggested that too much vitamin A (found in liver and cod liver oil) can increase the risk of osteoporosis.

Early menopause

If you have an early menopause, which is not treated with hormone therapy, this can lead to brittle bones because bones have started thinning earlier. For this and other reasons, if you have a significantly early or premature menopause, you are encouraged to consider HRT at least until around the age of 50 years (see Chapter 15).

Medical conditions and medications

If you have any of the following conditions, or are on these treatments, you may be at greater risk of brittle bones and should consider discussing the risk with your doctor:

Medical conditions

- early or premature menopause
- overactive thyroid

- taking too much thyroid medication to treat an underactive thyroid
- anorexia nervosa
- inflammatory bowel disease
- coeliac disease
- liver or kidney disease

Medication

- long-term steroids
- aromatase inhibitors
- chemotherapy
- other immune suppressant medications
- some antidepressants
- proton pump inhibitors
- lithium

Smoking and alcohol

Smoking and excess alcohol consumption are both linked to bone thinning and osteoporosis. Stopping smoking and reducing alcohol intake to within target limits is something that is also a positive change for many other aspects of your health in menopause, not just bone health. There are a number of established treatments to help with stopping smoking and addressing unhealthy drinking habits, but for these to work you must be self-motivated to make the change. If you would like help with these issues, you should consider speaking to your doctor or practice nurse.

Genetic factors

Genetic factors contribute to osteoporosis. Family history is important to consider. If a family member has osteoporosis or has suffered with bone fractures there is a greater chance that you may be predisposed. There is, however, a lot of variation in genetic risk of osteoporosis and environmental factors, discussed above, are likely to play a role in this variability.

> **KEY FACT**
>
> Research has estimated that approximately 62 per cent of an individual's risk of osteoporosis is due to genetic factors, while 38 per cent of the risk is due to lifestyle and environmental factors.

Additional factors affecting bone strength

If you are small and thin with a low weight you are generally considered at greater risk of bone thinning. In terms of ethnicity, if you are Caucasian or Asian you are at highest risk of osteoporosis after menopause. If you are African-American or Hispanic you will have a lower overall risk of osteoporosis.

PREVENTION

Prevention of the effects of bone loss in menopause requires an understanding of risks. You can then take action to reduce risk factors and seek expert advice if you find you do have a higher risk of brittle bones. It is also very important to do everything you can to prevent falling, which is a major cause of bone fractures in women after menopause. Hip fractures can be very serious as you get older, and pain and a decreased ability to carry out normal activities may occur following a broken bone.

Weight-bearing exercise such as walking, running, dancing and weight-training exercise are very good for bone health because these activities directly strengthen bone and they also build up muscles, which support your bones. Strong muscles will reduce your risk of falls and can also play a positive role in keeping pain from arthritis at bay. Frailty and weak muscles have the opposite effect. Regular physical activity is a win–win situation. We have already seen the important benefits of exercise for many other aspects of menopause in Chapter 4.

BONE-STRENGTHENING TREATMENTS IN MENOPAUSE

There are several medical treatments that can be used to reduce the loss of bone and/or increase bone formation in menopause. The most effective and natural treatment is oestrogen therapy, which is discussed in Chapter 14.

Drug treatments for osteoporosis (including bisphosphonates, denosumab, teriparatide, strontium, raloxifene and calcitonin) all have significant side effects and variable benefits and I will not discuss these treatments here. This is an individual discussion for you to have with your family doctor or specialist if you are confirmed to have osteoporosis and those medications are not used for prevention.

I have listed some of the most common risk factors for osteoporosis below. If you have any of these risk factors you should consider talking to your GP about whether you need a bone density scan:

- low calcium intake (less than 1000mg daily)
- low vitamin D (low sunlight exposure, no supplement)
- regular smoking
- alcohol above 14 units per week
- low exercise and activity

- family history of brittle bones
- medical problems, such as bowel, liver, kidney, coeliac and thyroid disease
- medications causing thin bones, such as steroids or aromatase inhibitors
- previous chemotherapy
- history of low weight/anorexia
- increased risk of falls for any reason
- premature menopause: before the age of 40

A quick recap

Your bone health in menopause is affected by many different factors. The most important action you can take to keep your bones healthy is ensuring you have the right amount of calcium and vitamin D in your diet or through supplements. Doing regular exercise, not smoking and limiting alcohol to within guidelines are important steps you can take to protect your bones.

Some factors are beyond your control and, if you feel you have more than one risk factor for brittle bones, you should discuss this with your doctor to see if you need further tests.

CHAPTER 13

Natural and Complementary Remedies

MANY OF MY patients ask about natural treatments to help support symptoms during menopause, so this chapter will outline the popular natural and herbal remedies that are available for menopause. However, this does not mean that I recommend them; as these treatments are not generally supported by strong research evidence, there are no guarantees of success. Natural and herbal supplements are not as closely regulated as licensed prescription medications and usually have less or no evidence for benefit or safety data from research studies. The amount of product, quality, safety and purity may vary between brands or even between batches of the same brand. That is not to say they are to be totally dismissed, and different options will suit different people.

It is important to inform your doctor before seeking treatment with unconventional therapies. Some alternative, homeopathic and herbal treatments contain active substances and guidelines from the UK's National Institute for Health and Care Excellence also state that many available herbal medicines have unpredictable dose and purity, and some herbal medicines have significant drug interactions, potentially resulting in unexpected side effects and risks. It is therefore important to have as much information as possible about potential side effects and interactions before you try something new. It is recommended that herbal supplements are stopped for two to four weeks before any planned surgery.

If alternative, natural and herbal remedies do work for you, they can still be considered (see safeguarding notes on page 175). Some women gain benefit from these treatments. There is no evidence that alternative or herbal treatments work for life-threatening diseases such as cancer and organ failure, and they should not be used as a substitute for established treatment in these diseases. It's worth noting that the jury is still out about how most alternative and herbal remedies work.

HERBAL REMEDIES

Phytoestrogens

These are plant-based oestrogen-like compounds found in a number of sources including soy, flaxseed and red clover. They are structurally similar to oestradiol, which is a natural human oestrogen. They cause oestrogenic effects by binding weakly to oestrogen receptors, but they do not appear to affect blood levels of oestrogen. Proposed benefits include reduction in hot sweats and flushes, and improved sleep. They are not currently recommended for patients with breast cancer due to lack of safety data.

Phytoestrogens can be consumed through natural food sources or supplements such as red clover extracts. Research studies of red clover show no consistent or conclusive evidence of benefit for hot flushes in menopause. Studies report few side effects and no serious health problems with use. Despite lack of evidence many women choose to take red clover for reducing hot flushes.

Black cohosh

Although some studies have found that black cohosh may help hot flushes, the evidence is mixed. In addition, there is a lack of long-term data on the safety of this supplement. It can cause some mild side effects, such as stomach upset, cramping, headache, rash, a feeling of heaviness and weight gain, among other symptoms. Recent research suggests that black cohosh does not act like oestrogen, as once thought. There are some concerns that black cohosh may be associated with liver damage.

St John's wort

This is a herbal remedy that is used for lifting mood. St John's wort contains active ingredients including hyperforin. It has been studied in randomised controlled trials of major depression and shown to be as good at treating mood as conventional antidepressants. It has not been studied for milder or atypical depression. It is important for women in menopause to know about this supplement because it is sometimes recommended for symptoms of menopause such as hot flushes and mood changes.

You must, however, be warned that St John's wort might cause serious interactions with some medications and I would not recommend taking it alongside any prescription medication. For example, in those people taking blood-thinning medication, St John's wort might reduce the medication effect and cause blood clots. Because of the risks, France has banned the use of St John's wort in products. In some countries, St John's wort is only available with a prescription.

St John's wort has been shown to relieve menopausal hot flushes, particularly in women with a history of, or at high risk of, breast cancer. But women on treatment with tamoxifen should not take St John's wort as it can make tamoxifen ineffective.

DHEA (dehydroepiandrosterone)

DHEA is a natural steroid hormone produced by healthy adrenal glands. Its roles include beneficial effects on sex drive, energy, motivation and body shape. It is not licensed in the UK for menopause. It is classed as a food supplement in the United States and is popular for its proposed general anti-ageing effects.

Dong quai

Dong quai has been used in Traditional Chinese Medicine to treat gynaecological conditions for more than 1,200 years. I have found only one randomised clinical study of dong quai to determine effects on hot flushes, and it was not found to be useful in reducing them. Dong quai should not be used by women with fibroids or blood-clotting problems such as haemophilia, or by women taking drugs that affect clotting, such as warfarin, as bleeding complications can result.

Evening primrose oil

Evening primrose oil is helpful for benign breast pain and has also been promoted to relieve hot flushes. But its effect may be similar to placebo (see page 175). Side effects include inflammation, problems with blood clotting and the immune system, nausea and diarrhoea. It has been seen to cause seizures in patients with schizophrenia who are taking antipsychotic medication. Evening primrose oil should not be used with anticoagulants or mood-regulating drugs.

Starflower oil

Starflower oil contains gamma linolenic acid. It has anti-inflammatory and antioxidant properties. It can help with menopause hot flushes and night sweats and can also help with breast tenderness, anxiety, mood swings and skin breakouts.

Ginseng

Research has shown that ginseng may help with some menopausal symptoms, such as mood, sleep and overall well-being. However, it has not been found to be helpful for hot flushes.

Kava

Kava may decrease anxiety, but there is no evidence that it decreases hot flushes. It is important to note that kava has been associated with potential damage to the liver.

Liquorice extract

Some data suggest that liquorice extracts decrease the frequency and severity of hot flushes and other menopausal symptoms. It should be noted that too much liquorice can be harmful and the small amounts contained in herbal remedies may interact with prescription medication.

Other alternative remedies

There are a lot of other natural remedies around. Evidence for these helping menopausal symptoms is scarce for most of them, such as probiotics and prebiotics (gut microbiome and mood), ginkgo biloba (flushes and memory), sage and wild yam.

Guidelines recommend that you look for the THR logo, standing for 'traditional herbal registration'. These products have been approved and you can be sure that the product has the correct dosage, is of high quality and has suitable product information.

The use of homeopathy may or may not work for you. It is your individual choice, but there is no scientific evidence to support its use.

With any alternative therapy or herbal product, it is of the utmost importance to read all the contraindications and side effects of any of these interventions, especially if you are currently on any prescription medication for any medical condition.

Herbal and natural remedies are generally considered alternative to conventional treatments. In contrast, a number of complementary therapies can be used alongside conventional treatments without interaction.

COMPLEMENTARY APPROACHES

Complementary therapies include acupuncture, reflexology, reiki, osteopathy, aromatherapy, magnetism and massage therapy. These therapies are now very popular in the Western world, despite scanty research evidence of benefit. There are several anecdotal reports and many people swear by these treatments for a number of ailments. It is possible that some of these treatments may work through a placebo effect (see below).

Research to unequivocally demonstrate benefits of complementary therapies would be difficult to undertake on a large scale because funding costs would probably be prohibitive. It is therefore unlikely that these will be licensed for menopause management anytime soon. Although they are unlicensed treatment options, they appear safe. For menopause symptoms, it therefore seems reasonable to consider such therapies as long as they do not represent too great a financial cost to the individual.

These therapies should not replace prescribed treatments that your medically qualified healthcare professional recommends because they are not generally used as standalone or alternative treatments for medical illness.

Micronutrient supplementation may also be considered complementary. From a well-being perspective, it is important to ensure that you optimise your intake of micronutrients (see Chapter 5).

Cognitive behavioural therapy

Cognitive behavioural therapy (CBT) – a psychological-based therapy that helps to challenge and change your unhelpful perceptions, thoughts and behaviours – should be considered a mainstream treatment rather than being an alternative therapy, but it is still generally considered as complementary. It has good independent evidence of benefit in managing menopause symptoms. It can be used prescriptively as a course of treatment, but is still not widely accessible to many women in menopause. For more information about CBT and mindfulness techniques please see Chapter 10.

THE PLACEBO EFFECT

Some alternative menopause treatments could potentially work through a placebo effect. Placebo treatments may make you feel better, but they will not cure any underlying disease. Placebo effect should not be discounted, as any symptom relief is valuable regardless of how it works as long as it is used safely within the strict parameters of individual health safeguards.

Placebo effects can improve symptoms from many illnesses by up to around 50 per cent. The way a placebo works is thought to be through the induction of neural brain effects, but more work needs to be done to expand our understanding of this mechanism. Neuroscience research is working towards this understanding. From what we currently understand, it appears that dopamine and endorphins (feel-good hormones) are mediators of placebo effects. These findings suggest that there may be a true benefit of placebo treatment for certain symptoms, particularly problems such as pain, fatigue and hormone imbalances, possibly through altering certain brain hormones. Provided they are safe, they are therefore reasonable to try for menopause symptoms because menopause is not a disease.

SAFEGUARDS

1. Always check for incompatibilities with any current medical conditions/prescription medications being taken. Read the label very carefully. If unsure, ask your doctor.
2. Seek products that are approved by the UK regulatory body (traditional herbal registration), display the THR logo and are sold in well-known and reputable outlets (not dodgy websites with exaggerated claims and high prices!).

3. Remember, just because a product is herbal or natural does not mean it is gentle or without side effects. These products can be very potent.
4. Be aware that there may be a greater incidence of placebo effect with herbal products, but if they help and cause no harm then some people may want to consider them.
5. As a medical specialist, I cannot personally endorse any herbal or homeopathic remedy without evidence-based research, just as I would not endorse non-regulated conventional medications.

A quick recap

There are many natural and herbal remedies that seem to help many women in menopause and, as long as they are safe and not too costly, they are fine to try. The mechanism of how they work is rarely understood and large studies testing them are not generally available. There are also many complementary therapies that work in ways we still don't fully understand and can be very helpful for menopausal symptoms. The choice here is yours, and you will need to take a view to see if they have helped after a trial to decide if you want to continue using them.

PART 3

Treatment Options When Self-Management Is Not Enough

CHAPTER 14

Sex and Intimacy

I N THIS CHAPTER I want to mention the unmentionables. Love can hurt through menopause, both physically during sex and psychologically because of tensions in the bedroom and beyond. It has only been very recently that our world has come to terms with openly talking about this topic.

It is important to create dialogues about vaginal symptoms and sexual health after menopause because they are significant issues for many of us. Most importantly, there are multiple actions and approaches that can improve sexual function and vaginal symptoms in menopause.

Whether it be with partners, healthcare professionals or other women in a similar situation, openness enables not only discussion about managing symptoms but also troubleshooting and finding solutions. It is also good to know you are not alone in the problems that you face and that there are solutions that can improve many aspects of life in the bedroom.

KEY FACT

Around a third of premenopausal women and half of older women report sexual problems, with lack of desire a major cause, so this is not just a menopause issue.

Menopause is different today compared with previous generations and you will have your own unique experience. Loved ones are also part of the journey and menopause can affect relationship dynamics today more than ever before. Armed with the right information and by using simple supportive actions, your relationships can flourish and strengthen during menopause.

RELIGHT MY FIRE

As a modern woman in today's busy world you are likely to be juggling many balls. You may be expected to be everything to everyone, including maintaining passion in the bedroom. As menopause hits, many symptoms can hijack your mojo and libido. My patients discuss a whole variety of concerns, although the common themes I hear fall into some discrete categories. Concerns may be about mechanics – physical symptoms – or they may be more about emotional context. Your concerns may be related to having too much on, being overcommitted and just feeling too jaded. Sometimes the attraction of an early night can be more about recharging and catching up on sleep than an evening of intimacy with your partner.

General symptoms

Vaginal and bladder symptoms can affect intimacy and are common as oestrogen levels fall in menopause. Vaginal moisture and lubrication are reduced after menopause and the vaginal wall becomes thinner. General symptoms can include:

- dryness
- itching
- discomfort
- pain
- difficulties with bladder control
- incontinence
- bladder infections (UTIs)

The experience varies. You may have few symptoms, but, in some cases, these symptoms can have extreme effects on quality of life and can also affect sexual function.

KEY FACT

Vaginal and bladder problems occur in up to 40 per cent of women after menopause but only about 25 per cent will ask for help.

In order to seamlessly maintain your physical relationship in the bedroom, some adjustments and understanding by both you and your partner are likely to be beneficial and will help to create an environment of mutual harmony rather than tension. Addressing physical symptoms as well as emotional and psychological self-care are all important factors to be considered for both you and your partner.

CASE HISTORY: VANESSA

Vanessa came to see me because she was experiencing what she knew were menopause symptoms. She was having some hot sweats and her periods were all over the place. But her main concern was her mood. She was usually a very placid person and she had noticed she was becoming irritable and snappy at home, which was most unlike her. She was also juggling a busy job and had just been diagnosed with diabetes. This had caused symptoms of extreme fatigue and Vanessa herself knew that the additional fatigue was probably adding to her irritability. Vanessa had excellent insight

---

into her symptoms but the biggest problem for her was her partner. He kept insisting that he thought she was bipolar and that she needed to see a psychiatrist. This made Vanessa feel more anxious and produced tension in the relationship. Their sex life suffered, not due to menopause symptoms but because they were just not getting on. Her partner's unhelpful comments and suggestions actually made Vanessa feel more irritable around him and everything was starting to get difficult.

Having assessed Vanessa, I knew she was clearly not bipolar. She was experiencing some mood changes related to menopause. These did not represent a new mental health concern. Although they were not severe, they were difficult for her partner to cope with because he was so used to her being calm, steady and stable. I explained to Vanessa that her partner was likely to be afraid of the new symptoms. He didn't understand them and didn't know where things were leading. In his mind, he was probably hoping that his comments might help her 'snap out of it'. He was unaware that his emotional and instinctive vocalisations were not only unhelpful but likely to worsen Vanessa's symptoms and drive them apart.

I explained to Vanessa that she needed to look at practical ways of improving her mood. She had already started on medication for diabetes and was feeling less exhausted. I explained that she needed to ensure self-care and try not to take on too much commitment, at least until her diabetes had stabilised and she was feeling better. I explained that some of Vanessa's symptoms may be relieved by HRT, but Vanessa did not want to pursue that, at least until she had sorted out her diabetes, and she also felt that if her partner could be a bit more supportive, things would be much better. Vanessa brought her partner to a subsequent consultation and I explained to both of them what Vanessa was experiencing and how her partner's support, with some small adjustments in his behaviour to her, could transform the situation. Both were relieved to feel they understood what was going on and what was needed going forward. Understanding the mood changes, and that they would be temporary and eased by his support, helped Vanessa's partner to be there for her. Both Vanessa's symptoms and her relationship gradually got back on track.

THE ROLE OF LOVED ONES

Being in a relationship when you go through menopause can certainly have its challenges. You may be more irritable with your loved ones and it can often be difficult for them to understand and accept symptoms looking from the outside in. You may feel emotional for no obvious reason, which can be hard to experience, and loss of sex drive can cause sexual tension. Relationships can be put under strain, and there are many stories of relationship break-ups during menopause. If you have concerns about this, NHS-recommended relationship counselling services near you can be found on the NHS website.

Partners and loved ones are important stakeholders in menopause and they need to understand your menopause too! There is certainly a need for compromise, mutual understanding and partnership. Psychological support from loved ones is helpful for all health issues because emotional stress can be reduced by simple strategies like talking things through. This can work like a talking therapy with your loved ones, who may not be your partner – they may be a close friend or family member. If emotional stress is reduced, well-being tends to improve. If you have a female partner and you are both going through menopause at the same time, you may still experience very different symptoms and so understanding their perspective will be really helpful.

When someone is on the outside of a symptom or illness they can instinctively want to solve the problem. If they can't solve it they can sometimes feel frustrated and then may say or do something that is unhelpful or even harmful. They don't mean to do that, it is just an automatic instinct. In fact, just being there for you, lending a listening ear and offering simple supportive words and gestures can make a real positive difference. Giving you a simple hug and saying, 'It must be really hard for you right now', 'I am here for you' or 'Let me help with some of your chores today to take the pressure off' are simple strategies that can defuse a toxic situation and bring you closer together. They are not instinctive and so learning to remember them at times of need is important.

In the following table I have listed some situations in which your partner's response can make a difference to how you feel – some of the scenarios may be familiar. I have provided two different responses for each situation and it may help to show your partner the table to help them understand that a simple change in their response could help support you, strengthen your connection and ease your symptoms burden.

When symptoms overflow

Some situational examples	Partner do's	Partner don'ts
You have a meltdown about something unimportant	Make you a hot drink. Ask what they can do to help reduce your stress levels	Laugh, say you are going mad or storm out

Some situational examples	Partner do's	Partner don'ts
You are too exhausted to go on a night out	Give you a hug, rearrange the date, explain they understand you are struggling, and it must be hard for you, discuss later how they can help you feel less exhausted	Get moody because this has affected their social life
You feel low	Offer to have a chat about your feelings, offer you a hug. Suggest you meet with a close friend, or do something you enjoy, to help lift your mood	Ignore your sadness. Tell you to snap out of it
You cannot sleep	Ask if they can do anything to help. Do not judge. Say it must be hard having so little sleep	Make comments like 'Your sleep's dysfunctional and disrupts mine', 'I always sleep fine when you are not around'
You are feeling low in self-esteem	Tell you they love you the way you are. Remind you of all your good qualities	Ignore you. Tell you that you need to lose weight

Some situational examples	Partner do's	Partner don'ts
You don't feel like sex, they do	Try not to get frustrated. Plan a date for sex another day, make it a date so you can both get in the mood together	Get angry and sleep in the spare room

MENOPAUSE NOW

Equality matters, whether it be in the workplace, kitchen or bedroom, regardless of your age. You can expect more adult life after menopause than you had before it. Maintaining sexual intimacy is an important consideration after menopause for many women and their partners. Vaginal symptoms, among many other factors, can be addressed and optimised to ensure your sexual experience remains positive and fulfilled.

LET'S TALK ABOUT SEX

If things get difficult in the bedroom it is important to be aware that you can seek help. Many women defer seeking help about vaginal symptoms and loss of libido because of embarrassment and consider it to be a topic off-limits. This needs to change because there are several treatments and strategies that can help.

I am not a sexual health expert but as an endocrinologist I have undertaken consultations about many different sexual problems related to menopause over several years. When the bedroom suffers it can affect other aspects of a relationship and quality of life. Sometimes one partner is more motivated than the other to keep intimacy going or get things back on track. For many couples, keeping the flame alight or reigniting it in menopause is important to both parties. I also acknowledge that for some couples this is not an issue and that's also fine. Every couple's priorities will be different.

Below I will discuss symptom troubleshooting and using different types of treatment in different contexts. This will hopefully help you and your partner to identify some positive changes you can make that could help your sex life.

In menopause, sex drive and intimacy can be significantly affected by physical factors such as discomfort, pain and reduced arousal. These can interlock with psychosexual factors that can impact on sexual function and desire. Contributory factors range from the physical changes in the vagina to your overall physical health, psychological well-being, cultural and religious beliefs, wider relationship issues, self-image, stress and lifestyle factors. Stress and mood disorders can reduce overall motivation and interest; they can affect sex drive at any age and across genders, adding a further dimension to physical menopausal factors and sexual function.

There are many different types of treatment for vaginal symptoms and new treatments are becoming available all the time. The treatment needs to be tailored to your individual needs, and can be hormone- or non-hormone-based medications or vaginal treatments as well as psychological treatments. A combination of approaches usually works best. Vaginal symptoms can be the initial trigger for sexual difficulties in menopause. They continue to be a largely hidden, untreated problem, even though treatment can make a positive difference. As we are living longer after menopause, these dialogues need to get going.

Sexual desire often triggers arousal. After menopause, desire, which is influenced by hormones, may no longer be the initial sexual stimulus for arousal. Instead, desire tends to follow arousal. Arousal therefore needs to be triggered first usually from cues, signals or suggestions by your partner or your own conscious decision to initiate intimacy or respond to your partner's approach. Spontaneity can be more difficult when life is busy, so a degree of shared planning can help manage both partners' expectations and result in a more satisfying sexual encounter.

MANAGEMENT OPTIONS

In general, management requires a combination of different approaches. Although you may not see a link, it is important to be aware that the lifestyle factors discussed in Part 2 are important supporting measures because they can improve your overall well-being, mood and energy, which can all help with sexual satisfaction. Investing time in the sexual side of your relationship rather than putting things off can also make a positive difference to the experience for both you and your partner.

A logical approach to managing vaginal and sexual symptoms in menopause is to treat symptoms early to prevent them escalating out of control. Keeping your vagina healthy by ensuring long-term moisture and lubrication at times of intimacy, and reducing your risk of UTIs, are all helpful steps. Washing your genital area with warm water before and after sex may reduce the risk of bacteria getting into the bladder and this may decrease the risk of UTIs. Emptying your bladder before and after sex may also help reduce the risk of a UTI.

If vaginal symptoms are well-managed, many women benefit in terms of improvement in sexual satisfaction. If there are complex issues beyond the vagina, additional treatments will be needed, which I will touch on below. However, please bear in mind that I am not a sexual health expert; for complex sexual health issues, it is best to seek specialist input.

Vaginal lubricants and moisturisers

Vaginal lubricants and moisturisers work in different ways, but are both important for vaginal health in menopause. The moisturisers are longer acting and will help with general symptoms of dryness and discomfort. Lubricants help at the time of intimacy. They are safe, easy to apply and effective for many women. Most do not require a prescription. They reduce vaginal dryness and pain in women with mild symptoms and help prevent trauma and infections.

Vaginal lubricants

Vaginal lubricants do not tend to have very long-lasting effects and aim to provide relief of dryness, trauma and discomfort during sex. A variety of vaginal lubricants is available in pharmacies with or without a prescription and they can be water-based, plant-oil-based, mineral-oil-based or silicone-based. Examples of vaginal lubricants include YES and Sylk.

Oil-based vaginal lubricants can break down latex condoms, and therefore the water-based alternatives are preferable if condoms are being used, if there is any risk of contracting sexually transmitted infections or pregnancy (which is not unheard of in perimenopause!).

Vaginal moisturisers

Vaginal moisturisers imitate natural secretions by rehydrating the wall lining of the vagina. Moisturisers are not only used specifically for painful intercourse, but also for general symptoms down below, such as itching, dryness, burning and the need to pass urine more often. The effect of moisturisers is longer lasting compared with lubricants, if used regularly. They are usually applied about twice a week. Most vaginal moisturisers contain water and a variety of fillers that mimic natural mucus. Available vaginal moisturisers include Replens, Regelle and Hyalofemme.

Hormone therapies

Hormone treatments are usually recommended if non-hormone lubricants and moisturisers have not been effective. Hormone replacement therapy (HRT) can improve vaginal symptoms and is a good option if you are suffering from a lot of other menopause-related symptoms as well as vaginal symptoms (see Chapter 15). When symptoms are predominantly vaginal or bladder-related, local vaginal hormone treatments are usually recommended first. Even if HRT is given, vaginal symptoms can require the addition of vaginal oestrogen to treat vaginal symptoms. Vaginal oestrogen can independently improve sexual function in women with symptoms.

Several vaginal oestrogen preparations are available, including creams, vaginal tablets and rings. Vaginal oestrogen treatment does not result in womb thickening, and progesterone treatment (which is needed if oestrogen is given by tablet or skin preparation) is not required to balance vaginal oestrogen treatment.

If treatment with oestrogen could be hazardous for you because you have had a hormone-driven cancer such as breast cancer, non-hormone treatments are usually preferred. Safety data regarding the safety of vaginal oestrogen therapy in breast cancer survivors are limited to about three-and-a-half years follow-up. Treatment for that duration appears safe in women treated with tamoxifen, but possibly not with aromatase inhibitors. As secondary breast cancer can occur many years or even decades after the primary, it will be difficult to give full reassurance about any hormone treatment in women who have had breast cancer.

There does not appear to be an increased risk of recurrence of womb cancer when HRT is used following treatment for womb cancer. There does not appear to be an increased risk of recurrence of previous ovarian cancer with either HRT or vaginal oestrogen therapy.

TSECs

There are a few new medications that have recently become available to help vaginal symptoms and reduce pain on intercourse. While they appear safe and low in side effects, and study results appear promising, their effectiveness will be judged with time.

These include ospemifene and lasofoxifene, a group of drugs called TSECs that include synthetic oestrogen (non-bioidentical) derived from horse urine.

Phytoestrogens

Phytoestrogens (e.g. red clover oil), may help with vaginal dryness and pain on intercourse and appear to be safe in terms of oestrogen effects in the uterus. However, it is still recommended that products containing phytoestrogens should ideally be avoided in women who have risk factors for taking oestrogen.

Vaginal laser treatment

This is a new treatment and not currently widely available. It may stimulate growth of the vaginal lining and may help vaginal symptoms. Only small studies on this treatment have been conducted to date, so it is a 'watch this space' treatment.

Androgens (testosterone) and DHEA (dehydroepiandrosterone)

Testosterone has an effect on the vagina and is important for sexual function. During menopause, testosterone levels can fall. Testosterone can be given as a treatment in skin gel form to help with sexual desire and arousal in menopause, usually in conjunction with HRT. There have been problems getting a licence for testosterone use in menopause. There are a number of products licensed for men, which are used in adjusted doses, supervised by menopause specialists, for reduced sexual desire and arousal in menopause. A newer preparation of testosterone gel designed specifically for female usage (AndroFeme) is available from Australia by special licence and aims to get a full licence in the UK sometime soon.

Early studies conducted in women suffering from vaginal atrophy symptoms due to treatment with aromatase inhibitors for breast cancer, using treatment with vaginal testosterone, have shown promising results and the treatment does not affect oestrogen levels in the blood. Vaginal testosterone therefore offers potential as a treatment for vaginal and bladder symptoms in menopause, and may be a good option for vaginal symptoms in the future, particularly if you are treated with aromatase inhibitors for breast cancer, but more studies are needed.

DHEA is an androgen (male hormone but also important for women) made by the adrenal gland. After menopause, DHEA is a major source of sex steroid hormones. A new vaginal treatment called prasterone, which is a vaginal preparation of DHEA (Intrarosa), appears to enhance natural production of both androgen and oestrogen in the vagina. It is now available in the UK (licensed in 2019) and has been shown to be effective for managing painful sex in menopause.

CASE STUDY: JULIE

Sexual problems during menopause can sometimes prove difficult to untangle from broader physical, psychosexual and relationship issues. Julie was 47 years old and had an early menopause after chemotherapy for breast cancer. She came with her partner to discuss her lack of sex drive. Julie had a very healthy lifestyle, a good diet and did lots of exercise. She had received cognitive therapy about her cancer diagnosis and had adjusted well. Overall her menopause was unproblematic apart from her lack of libido. Julie's partner was doting and really wanted their sex life to be maintained, as did she. Julie was using vaginal lubricants effectively and didn't have any significant vaginal symptoms. She just really wanted more enjoyment of sex and intimacy with her partner.

After considering many options and after discussions with the breast team, Julie had a trial of testosterone treatment but she didn't feel it helped her. When I probed further (the couple had been quite elusive about the intimacy issues initially and simply insisted that Julie's sex drive was low), a major issue for Julie was the frequency that her partner wanted to have sex. Julie felt keen to have sex once a week but her partner felt that was abnormal and he wanted to have sex almost every day.

It was clear that Julie and her partner were on different pages about how often they wanted to have sex and intimacy. Every couple will have different views on what suits them and frequency of intimacy may or may not change over time and after menopause, but this should be mutually agreeable. Julie did not specifically have a sexual problem, but having sex every day was just too much for her after menopause. Julie and her partner went for psychosexual counselling and found mutual ground.

Addressing and resolving broader psychological and psychosexual issues, through psychosexual counselling, can be very useful for a wide range of sexual problems and relationship difficulties. Both individual and couples therapy can be helpful. The goal is to empower couples to understand the nature and sources of their sexual problems and feel liberated to express sexual wants and needs.

Other approaches

Overall well-being has an impact on sexual health and therefore all the self-directed lifestyle approaches discussed in Part 2 will help support management of sexual health issues in menopause.

You may have heard of Viagra and be wondering if it might work for you as it helps sexual problems in men. Viagra is more of a plumbing treatment in men that improves blood flow to the penis. Viagra is not an aphrodisiac and it doesn't appear to help with female sexual function.

There are a couple of new drugs now approved for use in the US called flibanserin (Addyi) – a daily tablet – and bremelanotide (Vyleesi), which is given by injection before sex. They have been likened to a female Viagra but they don't work in the same way. These new drugs affect levels of brain chemicals to improve arousal. They don't improve the overall sexual experience and can have major side effects, and are not currently available in the UK.

For severe pain on intercourse there are likely to be several contributory factors, and spontaneous vaginal pain is usually complex. If it becomes chronic, vaginismus (severe pain on penetration) and vulvodynia (chronic vaginal pain with no clear-cut cause) are possible additional diagnoses contributing to symptoms. These can occur at any age, but are not very common. Perineal (down below) pain can affect sex and intimacy. Treatment may require specialist advice. Strategies can include vaginal dilators, pelvic floor physiotherapy, gynaecology surgical intervention and sometimes pain-management medications if the pain is permanent and has not responded to all other measures.

In the table below I have outlined various available treatments for different sexual problems in menopause. If you identify with any of the specific symptoms you can look into the different treatments available yourself or speak to your GP about treatment.

Treatments for sexual problems after menopause

Low libido/sex drive	• Relationship strategies to increase desire: couples time, date nights, flirting, venturing beyond the humdrum, stimulation

	• Psychosexual counselling, couples therapy • Consider changing offending medication (see below): antidepressants (switch to bupropion), blood pressure meds (adjust or reduce dose) • Testosterone replacement • Stress-management techniques, lifestyle measures
Vaginal dryness	• Regular sexual activity or stimulation (promotes vaginal health and blood flow) • Vaginal lubricants (for temporary relief of dryness before and during sex) • Vaginal moisturisers (for longer-term relief from dryness) • Vaginal oestrogen therapy in cream, ring or tablet form • Consider prasterone • HRT (reverses underlying atrophy and dryness, but generally reserved for women with bothersome hot flushes)
Arousal difficulties	• Topical treatments for vaginal dryness/ atrophy • Vibrator/sex toys • Psychosexual counselling, couples therapy • Bupropion sometimes used • Relaxation techniques, lifestyle measures

Orgasm difficulties	• Psychosexual counselling, couples therapy • Relaxation techniques, lifestyle measures
Painful sex	• Vaginal moisturisers and lubricants • Vaginal oestrogen • HRT • Prasterone • Psychosexual counselling, couples therapy • Vaginal dilators • Pelvic floor physiotherapy • Gynaecological surgical intervention • Pain management drugs if pain is permanent

PRESCRIPTION MEDICATION AND ISSUES WITH SEXUAL FUNCTION

If you are being treated with lots of prescription medications for other health issues it is important to understand that some medications can interfere with sexual function and you should ask your doctor if any of your prescribed medications could be negatively affecting your sexual function.

KEY FACT

Several antidepressant and other medications can negatively affect sex drive.

Most antidepressant medications have a negative effect on sex drive, arousal and orgasm. Bupropion is a unique type of anti-depressant that does not negatively affect sexual function. It is commonly used in the UK as a stop-smoking medication. Some reports suggest it may increase libido. It can therefore be considered as an option if you need an antidepressant, but have sexual function side effects with the one you are taking. Bupropion can cause nausea and other side effects, and there is currently not enough evidence to suggest that it should be used widely for menopause sexual dysfunction if antidepressants are not needed for other reasons.

A quick recap

Sexual problems are quite common during menopause and there are many different physical, hormonal, psychological and lifestyle factors that can contribute to your symptoms. It is important for you to feel able to talk about any problems that you have with your partner and, if necessary, with your doctor. There are many treatments and solutions available to improve symptoms. Understanding your own specific challenges can be half the battle and lead to sustainable solutions.

CHAPTER 15

Hormone Replacement Therapy (HRT)

YOU HAVE ESTABLISHED that your symptoms are due to menopause and you are wondering whether you should try HRT. It may seem like a difficult decision, but I find that my patients soon identify their preferred path, as long as they have all the information to hand. One thing that it is important for you to understand is that it is much better for your overall long-term health to keep menopause symptoms at bay and have a menopause transition that does not feel like a torture chamber!

MENOPAUSE NOW

There has never been so much high-quality research data available about the safety and risks of HRT. Many formulations now available are much safer than the long-available synthetic alternatives. You can therefore make a more informed decision than ever before about whether HRT is right for you.

REASONS TO CONSIDER HRT

- 'My life is very challenging right now; symptoms are getting on top of me and I need to be at the top of my game to manage everything and to be there for my loved ones.'
- 'I have an early menopause, before 51 years, so HRT will protect my bones and blood vessels.'
- 'I am having drenching sweats day and night – I cannot live like this.'
- 'I am exhausted and I simply cannot do all the things I need to do.'
- 'I cannot sleep and it feels like torture going to bed every night.'
- 'My mood has crashed and there is no other trigger except my hormone changes.'
- 'I cannot function at work because of brain fog and hot sweats.'
- 'I am so irritable I am driving my partner away.'
- 'I have no sex drive, my vagina is dry and on fire, and that is making me miserable.'
- 'My muscular aches and pains are so much worse than before, I don't want to move.'

These are just a few examples of reasons to consider treatment with HRT; there are many more depending on your individual circumstances. If your lifestyle is already healthy and your symptoms are troublesome, like those in the list above, then a trial of HRT is a good idea and the benefits are likely to outweigh any risks.

HRT has a multitude of benefits. It helps with all menopausal symptoms, in particular sweats and flushes, mood changes, insomnia, vaginal and bladder symptoms, and sexual function. It also strengthens bones. HRT appears to protect against heart and blood vessel disease in women who do not already have these diseases and are under 60 years of age, so it is particularly important for women with early or premature menopause.

Provided that there are no overriding dangers or concerns, you should preferably start a trial of HRT early in your menopause journey. Early treatment will prevent symptoms from progressing and becoming more difficult to get under control later (the so-called 'crescendo effect'). It is not necessary or appropriate to be a martyr and suffer in silence – you suffering with severe symptoms is likely to have a negative impact, not only on your life and health, but also on those around you. Remember, self-care benefits your loved ones too.

On the other hand, if you are thinking, 'It doesn't seem to be that bad, although I have noticed some symptoms,' then the lifestyle toolkit in Part 2 should be your new best friend. I would urge you to implement the lifestyle measures detailed in Part 2 as part of any other treatment approach you choose, including HRT. Menopause needs a holistic and multifaceted focus. If lifestyle measures are optimised before menopause symptoms escalate, the symptom burden may be lessened and any additional intervention is likely to be more effective, including HRT. Also, coming off HRT at a later date will be easier if your lifestyle has been optimised.

If you feel that you are coping well with lifestyle measures, your quality of life is good and the prospect of HRT does not attract you, then there is no need to pursue it. This is your decision. The main exception to this recommendation is if you have had an early or premature menopause, in which case most menopause specialists would recommend treatment at least until natural menopause age – around 51 years. Another issue that can sway a decision about HRT is if you have osteoporosis. In this situation, if it is deemed safe and if you have some menopause symptoms, HRT is the best and safest bone-building treatment to strengthen your bones long-term.

If you have severe menopausal symptoms it is logical to take HRT, at least for a while. It is usually very safe for the first few years of treatment. There appear to be small risks associated with longer-term treatment, several years after natural menopause. More modern regimens, which tend to contain a form of oestrogen that is identical to natural human oestrogen (body identical), particularly in skin patch or skin gel forms, appear safer. Tablet oestrogen has to be broken down in the liver and the by-products can affect blood clotting. All tablet oestrogen preparations (combined pills and HRT) therefore increase background blood clot risk.

The newer progestogens used in HRT (which are needed for HRT unless you have had a hysterectomy) now tend to have less problematic side effects in the more modern combined preparations, compared to older preparations. The synthetic progestogens are still associated with some side effects and appear to be linked with a small increase in overall risks, when used continuously for several years.

The safest progesterone preparation is one that is identical to human progesterone. This was historically difficult to manufacture in tablet form, but a micronised form of progesterone has now been available as a licensed preparation for several years and has not been shown to result in any excess risks to date, with good research data available for up to five years' treatment. It also does not appear to increase the risk of blood clots.

Another point I often make to my patients who are unsure about HRT is that trying it for a short time, to see what the beneficial impact is and what side effects you experience, cannot do you any harm (unless you have major risk factors). You will know whether it can make a positive difference to your symptoms after only two to six weeks of treatment. And if it does not pass your test then you can stop knowing that you gave it a try.

KEY FACT

Progesterone is naturally produced by the body. Progestogen is a term given to a synthetic alternative. Natural progesterone has some health benefits, but synthetic progestogens have some side effects and longer-term risks.

TYPES OF HRT

All reputable hormone specialists in the UK and all NHS GPs will prescribe licensed preparations for HRT wherever possible. We now know that there are different pros and cons to different regimens. We have all the safety data at our fingertips for these licensed products. We know that even if you are treated with HRT for several years the overall risks are small and need to be balanced with the quality-of-life benefits that they bring to you.

In the past, HRT was mainly made from synthetic hormones and there have been a lot of problems with those causing the various health issues linked with HRT when used long-term, such as increased risks of blood clots, heart and blood vessel diseases, and breast cancer.

Licensed body-identical or bioidentical hormones are identical to your natural hormones and these are now widely available to use as HRT and appear safer. They are available in licensed preparations and doses that now have robust safety data available and so these preparations should be offered to you if you wish to have them.

Licensed bioidentical HRT may also be recommended if you have risk factors or problems with synthetic HRT preparations. An oestrogen skin patch or skin gel combined with tablet micronised progesterone appears to be the safest option if you have an increased risk of blood clots.

Bioidentical regimens can sometimes cause erratic bleeding, occasional unexpected side effects and can be slightly more cumbersome regimens to follow in a busy life. They usually involve continuous skin patch or skin gel oestrogen along with natural progesterone in tablet or pessary form, either continuously or cyclically.

If you decide that HRT is right for you, you will need to decide, with the help of your doctor, which type. There are many regimens, so understanding the whys and hows helps you home in on what will be best suited to you.

A NOTE OF CAUTION: COMPOUNDED BIOIDENTICAL HRT

These products are increasingly being prescribed by private practitioners who are not menopause specialists. They are not licensed medications and are not available on the NHS. They are effectively 'home-made to order'. You may think that sounds good, but those products do not come with safety warnings – not because they are 'natural and therefore safe' but because they are totally unlicensed and unregulated and safety is unknown. These products are promoted as being 'individualised'. This is misinformation. Any harm coming to women using these preparations is difficult to trace because there is no robust way of reporting harm arising from unlicensed drugs. Nonetheless, some studies looking at harm from these preparations have suggested that they can result in an increased risk of womb cancer and also blood clots.

It will be clear to you that you are being prescribed compounded bioidentical hormones because they are prescribed by very commercial, highly advertised clinics and the medication they give you will look like something tailor-made for you.

Cyclical HRT (oestrogen/oestrogen with progesterone in rotation)

If you are still having regular or irregular periods, or have had at least one bleed in the preceding 12 months, you will need a cyclical HRT regimen. This usually entails a preparation that contains oestrogen continuously, but progestogen/progesterone is added, usually for about two weeks per month, to keep your womb healthy and promote regular bleeding. You cannot have a 'non-bleed' preparation until you are at least a year out from your last natural period because if you take this when you are perimenopausal and still producing some oestrogen from your ovaries you can get erratic bleeding.

Cyclical HRT comes in tablets, skin patches and combinations of skin patches, skin gels and tablets.

Continuous HRT

These preparations can be used if you have not had a natural bleed for more than a year. They can also be used in younger perimenopausal women who have a progestogen coil (Mirena or Kyleena) that prevents bleeding.

These regimens should not result in any bleeding. They generally contain oestrogen and a low-dose progestogen in combination, in either tablet or skin patch form. With the progestogen coil, oestrogen patches, gel or tablets can be used. You can also take a combination of skin patch or skin gel oestrogen with tablet progesterone.

Oestrogen-only

This is suitable if you have had a hysterectomy. In general, you won't need progesterone (with the exception of the first year after hysterectomy for severe endometriosis). Oestrogen can be given as tablets, skin patches or gels.

Implants

Some gynaecologists still use implants after hysterectomy. Oestrogen and sometimes testosterone implants are used. Some women, particularly younger women who have had a total hysterectomy, like these implants because they are only needed every few months and you can forget about hormones in between treatments. However, something called 'tachyphylaxis' can sometimes occur with implants. This means that higher doses can be needed to get the same effects and oestrogen levels can sometimes be very high. This is obviously a concern both in terms of potential risks of very high oestrogen levels and the fact that, if a new breast cancer occurs, there is no easy way of removing the implant and shutting down the oestrogen quickly.

BLEEDING WITH HRT

During perimenopause, before your ovaries have completely stopped working, production of oestrogen can be erratic. This can result in thickening of the womb lining and irregular bleeding. HRT given in perimenopause is a cyclical type that aims to give you a monthly bleed by giving you a combination of hormones sequentially. This can regulate bleeding and should result in a monthly bleed reproducing a period.

If you have heavy, erratic or painful bleeding going through perimenopause, or if the bleeding makes you anaemic, a good option to consider is a progestogen hormone intrauterine device (IUD) coil, which your doctor or gynaecologist may recommend. This can usually stop bleeding altogether in perimenopause and protects the womb lining. If you have a hormone coil this also provides contraception. With a hormone coil if you suffer from menopausal symptoms then you can have oestrogen gel, patches or tablets to treat your symptoms without adding in any more progestogen treatment (because the coil has covered this).

Once you are at least one year out from your last natural period you can usually change to a continuous combined preparation of oestrogen and progesterone. By this time your womb lining has usually become thin so you do not tend to need the cyclical proges-terone to induce a bleed and the low-dose continuous preparations of oestrogen and progesterone will usually prevent the lining from thickening again. After the change in treatment there may be some spotting at the beginning, but this usually settles completely after a few months and then it should not result in any bleeding at all.

If you don't have bleeding with your HRT and then have an unexpected bleed this will need to be investigated to exclude any womb thickening or other womb abnormality. You will be referred to a gynaecologist, who will usually arrange a pelvic ultrasound and hysteroscopy (looking inside your womb with a camera, through your vagina), which can be done as a day case without anaesthetic. It is relatively common to get unscheduled bleeding on HRT and it's usually nothing to worry about, but it must be checked out just in case it is the start of something serious.

BREAST CONCERNS

Breasts can be engorged and sore in younger women in response to hormone changes of the monthly cycle, and the same can happen with women on HRT. Oestrogen is an active hormone in breast tissue and HRT can result in changes in the breasts including soreness and lumpiness. Knowing your own breasts is important because then you will notice if there is a sudden change and you can ensure you get checked out quickly.

One in eight women will develop breast cancer in their lifetime and more than 55,000 women are diagnosed each year in the UK alone. Statistics dictate that while HRT is used, there will inevitably be women who are diagnosed with breast cancer while they are taking HRT. That in itself does not mean that the HRT caused the cancer.

There is a small excess risk of breast cancer in women treated with combined HRT over several years after natural menopause age (51 years) compared with women who have never taken HRT. However, there are several other risk factors for breast cancer that we don't always give thought to.

Breast cancer risk

A study published in *The Lancet* journal in 2019 explained that, overall, 3 out of every 50 women are expected to develop breast cancer between the ages of 50 and 69 years, and that the use of combined HRT for 5 years, starting at 50 years, would result in one extra breast cancer case (between the ages of 50 and 69) for every 50 women treated. The authors demonstrated that women appear to remain at increased risk for more than 10 years after they stop taking HRT.

Overall research data therefore suggest that combined HRT can increase the overall risk of developing breast cancer. These are statistical risks. Each individual woman will have her own unique risk and benefit balance with HRT. A woman with a family history of breast cancer is likely to have a higher overall risk. Other important lifestyle factors also have a significant influence on breast cancer risk. If a woman maintains a healthy body weight, does not smoke, does two-and-a-half hours or more of physical activity per week and limits alcohol to 14 units or fewer per week, her risk of developing breast cancer will be significantly reduced.

It is always difficult to apply statistics to individual cases. Decisions about HRT need to be individual, balancing risks, benefits and personal preference. Whether or not HRT is used, positive lifestyle measures (discussed in the lifestyle toolkit in Part 2) can significantly reduce your risk of breast cancer and improve your overall well-being during menopause with no downside or risk.

Understanding risks helps with decision-making. If your quality of life is being affected by severe menopausal symptoms, the benefits of HRT may well outweigh the risks.

HOW LONG TO TAKE HRT

There is no time limit on HRT treatment and you should never be forced to stop treatment if you continue to gain benefit, wish to continue and are aware of the potential risks.

It is important in the throes of a difficult menopause transition to ensure that you have the choice to use HRT, which can certainly be life-changing in many situations. It is also important to acknowledge that risks may increase over several years and as you get older, and that regular review is required to reassess whether treatment is still needed years later and if your symptoms have settled down.

Although the natural HRT preparations are much safer, starting in your forties or fifties, their longer-term risks are unknown. Previous large-scale studies have suggested that the greatest risks of HRT are associated with longer duration of treatment and older age, particularly after the age of 60. No studies have suggested that lifelong HRT is safe or indeed necessary for most women.

A review of new evidence in 2019 relating to the 2015 National Institute for Health and Care Excellence guideline on menopause management looking at long-term benefits and risks of HRT showed no new data necessitating changes in guidance, with different studies showing increased risk, no benefit and improved risk for various outcomes with long-term HRT. New evidence relating to diabetes and dementia risk with HRT was found to be inconsistent and inconclusive. Therefore, the main reason to take HRT is for symptoms, well-being and quality-of-life benefits.

KEY FACT

There is no current conclusive peer-reviewed evidence suggesting that HRT should be used for preventing any diseases long-term, with the exception of treating osteoporosis for fracture prevention in the presence of menopause symptoms.

HRT appears safe for up to five years of treatment. After 10 years of treatment, and after the age of 60, overall risks appear to increase slightly, but this depends on individual risk, type of HRT and the balance of risk with the symptom benefit that you gain.

It is usually possible to gradually tail off treatment without any ill effects after a period of years, once your underlying hormone fluctuations stabilise and symptoms spontaneously resolve. If menopause was very early, tailing off treatment is usually deferred at least until around the average menopause age (51 years).

If you have had several years on treatment with HRT and are unable to wean off because of rebound symptoms, you should be supported to make a decision to continue treatment after discussing this with your doctor. As long as you are informed about potential risks, you should be supported in a decision to continue HRT regardless of your age if that is your wish.

During long-term HRT treatment, at any age it is important to review safety and risk at each doctor's appointment. Factors that your doctor will need to review include whether the type and dose of HRT is still right, that your blood pressure is under control, that mammograms are up to date, that no unscheduled vaginal bleeding has occurred and that any new symptoms or newly diagnosed conditions are taken into consideration.

How to come off HRT

If you are otherwise well and want to try to come off HRT, the best time to consider tailing down HRT is when menopausal symptoms are under control and when you have implemented robust lifestyle measures that will be your long-term substitute for hormone therapy.

In general, it is not a good idea to withdraw HRT abruptly. The sudden drop in hormones can cause withdrawal symptoms and destabilise well-being. One situation that can result in needing to abruptly stop HRT is when a new breast cancer is diagnosed during treatment with HRT. This is a situation where additional non-hormone treatment can be very useful to counteract rebound symptoms.

If treatment is gradually reduced, your body has time to readjust to the slowly changing status quo. The transition to the postmenopause, post-HRT phase is then seamless and tolerated much better for most women.

If and when you feel ready, I usually recommend an attempt at slowly tailing down treatment over 12–18 months. If you tail down but get to a lower dose that you don't feel able to go below, then you can just stick at that level for a while and have another go at tailing further after a few months. Tailing off HRT is not a precise science and the timing and success will be different for everyone. The dose changes during tailing will depend on what preparation you are on and should be supervised by your doctor.

If you are in the middle of major life events, stresses or trauma it is likely that tailing down HRT will be challenging and may result in a destabilisation of symptoms, so I would recommend deferring tailing treatment until life is more stable.

For most women making the choice to tail off HRT, symptoms do not return after tailing off HRT and, if they do, they are usually much milder. Menopause symptoms usually gradually settle over time even in women who do not take HRT.

PROBLEMS AND RISKS ASSOCIATED WITH HRT

Treatment with HRT can be problematic. You may develop complications during treatment, and some women may experience side effects, which can occur even with the licensed body-identical preparations that are the most natural forms and available on NHS prescription. You may simply not gain benefit and relief of symptoms despite HRT. You may choose not to take it due to underlying health risks or conditions, such as oestrogen-driven cancers. You may choose not to go down the HRT route at all.

If you want HRT but have significant risk factors, you should be provided with all the information to enable you to make your own balanced judgement. If you are at greater risk of harm from HRT, it is not enough for a healthcare professional to simply re-assure you that you can take it if you want to. You can only truly make an informed choice if you understand your own individual risks and benefits.

Blood clots

In general, a woman with a history of blood clots should not take tablet forms of oestrogen HRT because of the increased blood clot risk. However, such women can safely take oestrogen through a skin patch or gel because these do not increase blood clot risks. The type of progestogen used in this context is also an important consideration as synthetic progestogens may also increase blood clot risks.

Hormone-driven cancers

Cancers of the breast and womb can be driven by oestrogen. About 80 per cent of breast cancers have oestrogen receptors and can therefore be fed by oestrogen. Universal recommendations are therefore to avoid any hormone treatment after diagnosis with this type of breast cancer. This is because even when the cancer appears to be cured, a proportion of women will later develop secondary breast cancer. That is why adjuvant cancer therapy is continued for up to 10 years in many women after hormone receptor-positive breast cancer. Oestrogen treatment could inadvertently feed any cancer cells that have not been dealt with by initial treatment and risk the cancer coming back.

There are no robust safety data to reassure women who have been diagnosed with breast cancer that HRT is safe. Breast cancer is an unusual cancer in that it can return several years or even decades after the primary cancer appeared to be cured. Recurrence can occur in women who have had early-stage breast cancer as well as more aggressive breast cancers. It is unlikely that data on safety of short-term HRT treatment in this context can be truly reassuring.

Vaginal oestrogen has been used more frequently than standard HRT after breast cancer. This is likely to be safer because it is not acting all over the body, only in the vagina (see page 190)

In early-stage womb cancer, particularly in younger women who are put into menopause early by the treatment, the benefits of HRT may outweigh the risks, and treatment generally appears safe. The decision about having HRT after womb cancer should therefore follow a detailed discussion between the woman and her specialist to balance the risks and benefits and allow an informed decision.

There are no data to suggest an increased risk of recurrence of previous ovarian cancer with HRT. However, new ovarian cancer risk appears to be increased slightly in women treated with HRT.

Age

Age should not in itself be a barrier to HRT, although as you get older and further away from natural menopause you may develop other health problems that can make HRT less safe, such as heart and blood vessel disease or stroke. Also, as menopause symptoms settle over time, the benefits of treatment as we get older may not outweigh the risks.

NO HRT, NO PROBLEM

Women may choose not to take HRT for a number of reasons:

- If you have risk factors you may not feel comfortable taking HRT.
- If you are a breast cancer survivor it is generally advised that, ideally, you should not take HRT because of the potential risk of triggering a recurrence that could induce stage 4 incurable secondary disease.
- If you have had an unscheduled bleed on HRT and are found to have a thickened womb, your gynaecologist may advise you to tail off or stop HRT.
- You may have tried a number of HRT regimens and just didn't get on well with them.
- It is also possible that you may not achieve symptom relief with HRT.

- You may choose not to take HRT because you would rather allow your body to rebalance naturally using lifestyle approaches.

There is no study suggesting that lifelong HRT is safe for everyone, no matter what type of HRT is used. For these and other reasons it is important for all of us to look beyond HRT for management strategies to help with symptoms long-term.

Since media interest in menopause has started to escalate, the main focus has tended to be short-term success stories with HRT. The stories of women who can't tolerate HRT, who have complications with it or who optimise their own menopause experience with self-directed lifestyle measures don't tend to make news. You therefore need to be cautious and discerning when you see headlines because they can sometimes give a view that is not necessarily representative.

Lifestyle measures such as stress management, regular exercise, healthy sleep practices, good nutrition and maintaining a healthy weight, along with not smoking and moderating alcohol intake, are all powerful at reducing the risk of heart disease, many cancers, dementia, diabetes, high blood pressure and other health issues at any age. They also have huge quality-of-life benefits with no associated downside or risk. There are also many natural supplements, complementary therapies and non-hormone medications that may help stabilise your symptoms and all these measures can also be used if and when you decide to tail off HRT.

I see many women who manage to successfully discontinue HRT and many who have not used HRT who are thriving in menopause using lifestyle measures successfully. Lifestyle measures that help with menopause symptoms also have a capacity to reduce the stress load on the body (known as allostasis – see page 122). These measures effectively keep the body's balance and adrenal stress response healthy. After menopause we rely on the adrenal glands for the majority of sex hormone action in the body. It seems logical that healthy adrenals after menopause will be better able to compensate for the deficiency of ovarian sex hormones. That may in part explain why chronic stress and poor lifestyle tend to make the menopause experience worse whether HRT is used or not.

A quick recap

You need to understand your own individual pros and cons and risks and benefits of HRT, so that you can make an informed choice about whether to give it a try. If you feel that, despite your best efforts, your quality of life is being impacted by menopausal symptoms, you should speak to your doctor about a trial of HRT. If you do not have any major risks, you should not avoid HRT if symptoms are overflowing and affecting you and your loved ones. This is not just about self-care, but all your important roles in life. If you don't think you need HRT or don't feel it is safe for you there is no need to take it. Either way you can change your mind.

HRT is helpful to many women, particularly during a challenging life and when menopausal symptoms are at their worst. Equally, many women do manage menopause successfully without HRT.

HRT is not a substitute for lifestyle measures in menopause. The lifestyle measures outlined in Part 2 should be the cornerstone of symptom management, and HRT and other medications should be considered as accessories that some women will depend on and others will not want or need.

PART 4

Other Menopause Considerations

CHAPTER 16

Menopause at Work

Your employer should be made aware that menopause is a normal stage in life and that, in the main, with the right support, it will not, or very slightly, impact your ability to function normally at work and that symptoms are usually time-limited. We know that approximately three out of four women experience some symptoms and more openness about this is needed. However, for approximately 25 per cent of us, symptoms will be bothersome enough to need therapeutic intervention in our workplace, ranging from general understanding to workplace adjustments. Employers should not be misled into believing that menopause is an illness or that all women will need special treatment.

The number of menopausal women in work is likely to keep rising because we are all expected to work for longer before retirement; in the UK the state pension age has been gradually increasing for both men and women in recent years, and will reach 67 years by 2028.

It is true that menopause can have effects that may interfere with various aspects of your work function. Depending on symptoms, you will be better able to meet your full potential at work during menopause if you get the right support from your employer. Research has linked severity of menopausal symptoms with women intending to leave employment. This is now widely recognised and companies are increasingly starting to take action, looking into how they can support their employees suffering from menopausal symptoms and create menopause-friendly working environments. Research is also being conducted to look at organisational policies that will facilitate workplace culture change.

MENOPAUSE NOW

Women over the age of 50 are the fastest growing demographic in the UK workforce, with 4.4 million women aged 50–64 in work. The number has risen by 50 per cent in the last 30 years. According to the Faculty of Occupational Medicine, nearly 8 out of 10 menopausal women are in work. This means that there are a lot of women juggling work and menopause, as well as the rest of their lives.

It is clear from the statistics that menopause is likely to have an increasing impact on workforce logistics going forward. In order to maintain equality and diversity, and prevent discrimination, as well as ensuring staff retention and maintaining productivity, some MPs are calling for corporate reforms. The Chartered Institute of Personnel and Development (CIPD), the conciliation service ACAS and UNISON have all produced guidance on how employers and managers should support employees in menopause.

Providing you, as an employee, with information about menopause, as well as educating managers and human resources personnel, are crucial starting points to improve the menopause workplace experience as well as productivity.

For all stakeholders, shaking off the taboo and enabling an understanding of how menopause can affect work performance, how work environments can affect menopause symptoms and how reasonable adjustments can help with maintaining successful work roles will benefit all parties.

> **KEY FACT**
>
> There have already been employment tribunals successfully upheld in the UK for women in menopause based on gender discrimination in 2012 and disability discrimination (under the Equality Act of 2010) in 2018.

RESPONSIBILITY OF THE EMPLOYER

There are many, often interlocking, menopause factors that can impact on work performance. Many can be mitigated in the context of a sympathetic, supportive work environment and modest reasonable adjustments. The menopause-friendly workplace, which is already being adopted by some progressive organisations, could therefore be transformational with respect to productivity, inclusivity and organisational success. This type of workplace culture change could facilitate more women to be able to access and contribute diversely to a wider range of employments that have historically been under-represented by women. This could improve equality and diversity in a large swathe of organisations that are currently male-dominated.

Factors that impact on work performance include hot sweats, flushes, poor sleep, mood issues, anxiety, stress, brain fog, fatigue, headaches/migraine, recurrent urine infections, muscular and joint pains, heavy periods, anaemia, and non-menopause-related life events and health issues. These can all have differing impacts on work performance but can also be interlinked. It is important to note that you yourself may not be fully aware to what extent menopause may be contributing to your symptoms. While the topic remains off-limits, menopause is likely to remain under-reported as a cause for workplace difficulties and leaving employment.

It is very important for all line managers to have an understanding of the potential impact of menopause on employment to prevent even inadvertent discrimination from occurring, due to non-recognition of menopause as a health factor affecting work roles. If there is recognition that menopause may be affecting your work performance and capability, a referral to occupational health (where this is available) would be advised. Employers have a duty of care to do this. For smaller companies, obtaining evidence-based information, and liaising with suitable outside agencies where necessary, should be undertaken to ensure appropriate and timely supportive action.

There are some simple generic workplace adjustments, such as raising awareness to foster a menopause-friendly work environment and having health and well-being champions to enable openness and reduce stigma, and other more tailored strategies that can be implemented to support employees. The earlier problems related to menopause are recognised and addressed, the less negative impact on work performance the symptoms are likely to have.

Not all workplaces will be able to offer flexible working or shortened hours, so a conversation between you and your line manager to see what can be adjusted to support you within the scope of that organisation would be beneficial.

As you go through menopause you do not want to feel ill. You want to work efficiently and be valued by your employer. Providing reasonable adjustments for long-term health conditions, including menopause, should be considered mandatory by employers based on the Equality Act of 2010. By taking menopause difficulties seriously, treating them as an occupational health concern and providing you with appropriate reasonable adjustments, your job satisfaction and commitment are likely to be improved, your sickness is likely to be reduced and ultimately you will be less likely to leave your job. Recent guidance by CIPD supports these recommendations.

Responsibility of healthcare professionals

There is also an important role for primary care doctors and nurses in supporting you as an employed women suffering from menopausal symptoms. You may require prescription medication to help your symptoms, including the option of HRT. Having a supportive practitioner who understands menopause and can support the necessary management approach is vital.

TROUBLESHOOTING YOUR MENOPAUSE SYMPTOMS AT WORK

Many of the symptoms and troubleshooting solutions for managing menopause at work will be interchangeable. Therefore it is important to look synergistically at solutions in the context of your overall symptoms. I will discuss each symptom separately here, but some solutions will inevitably overlap.

This practical guide is based on my own clinical understanding of menopause and decades of experience advising employees and employers about strategies to help maintain employment in the context of complex symptoms. There is a lack of research data on this subject, but my recommendations are allied with existing evidence and recent guidance.

Sweats and flushes

Significance/impact: These can be embarrassing, awkward, debilitating and physically distressing. They can be very random and unpredictable. They can result in agitation. They can feel like being suffocated; therefore in the wrong environment, with no exit option, symptoms can become very distressing and trigger anxiety and other symptoms.

Self-management: Wear layers of clothing that can be removed easily. Avoid wool, silk and synthetic fabrics. Portable or desk fans can be really helpful. Have a plan of action for when a sweat begins, for example being able to remove layers, and go somewhere cool quickly. Plan your day – try to avoid rushing or being late. Avoid spicy food and have iced drinks rather than hot ones.

221

Consider asking your GP about medication including HRT if these measures don't work.

Brain fog

Significance/impact: You may have reduced focus and concentration and this can impact meetings and face-to-face communication, and can slow your work performance and reduce productivity. These factors can also affect your deadlines.

Self-management: Avoid eating a high-sugar breakfast, which can result in blood sugar dips and loss of focus some hours later. Optimise B vitamins and zinc (through diet or a supplement). Plan your day and avoid last-minute preparation/rushing. Have meals containing slow-release carbs to keep your blood sugar level steady through the day, because blood sugar dips can affect concentration. HRT can help brain fog.

Fatigue

Significance/impact: Fatigue can impact on your punctuality and cause slower work performance, reduced concentration, reduced productivity and missed deadlines. It can also affect mood.

Self-management: Ensure you have regular meals, including breakfast, and include slow-release carbs to limit blood sugar dips through the day, as these can cause fatigue. Try to keep a sleep routine, and try not to nap or minimise napping during the day. Try to get some exercise by walking in the fresh air during your lunch break; this can help with afternoon focus. Flexible working or working from home intermittently may be supported by your employer.

Low mood

Significance/impact: This can affect your communication and work relationships, self-esteem, reduce your motivation at work, reduce productivity and cause sleep disruption and fatigue. It can also be disruptive for your home environment.

Self-management: Mindfulness approaches. Ask your GP about CBT. Some larger employers have in-house provision or out-sourced mental health support provision. Try to increase exercise as it can boost well-being. Try to eat a healthy, balanced diet. HRT may help these symptoms. Discuss with your employer a support plan of necessary adjustments to help you stay in, or return to, work. Having a plan of management may lower anxiety associated with low mood.

Headaches/migraine

Significance/impact: Especially in perimenopause, this can be debilitating and result in sickness absence if attacks are severe or cause significant reduced work function during an attack if this occurs at work.

Self-management: These debilitating symptoms usually settle down with time once menopause is established. Try to identify and avoid any specific triggers, which may include stress or certain foods and drinks. Speak to your doctor about whether medication is needed.

Stress and anxiety

Significance/impact: Can contribute to poor concentration, brain fog, poor focus, reduced productivity, reduced confidence and self-esteem, and can affect work relationships. Can be debilitating during formal work presentations and meetings. If not addressed could lead to panic attacks and/or depression and sickness absence.

Self-management: Try mindfulness-based stress-management techniques (MBSR). CBT sometimes helps. Discuss these with your GP. Exercise also helps with stress. Try to ensure you are not overcommitted at work. Discuss reasonable work adjustments with your line manager.

Insomnia

Significance/impact: Reduced concentration at work, fatigue and low mood.

Self-management: Keeping a sleep routine is helpful even if it doesn't seem to resolve insomnia quickly. Sleep issues usually take a long time to change. If you are woken by night sweats or pain discuss treatment with your GP. If you work different shift patterns you can ask your employer if they can limit your shift changes.

UTIs (urine infections)

Significance/impact: Physically distressing symptoms, may need time off sick to recover. These can be recurrent in menopause.

Self-management: Vaginal moisturisers and lubricants can be very helpful. Attend to female hygiene. Ask your GP about treatments that could address the drop in oestrogen levels that can trigger recurrent UTIs.

Muscular/joint pains

Significance/impact: Hand joint pain can be worsened by a computer-based job. Physical work roles can worsen long-term injuries/back problems. Pain can worsen sleep and fatigue. Pain medications can cause many side effects and affect your well-being and work performance.

Self-management: Regular physical activity and movement are almost always helpful. Physiotherapy and anti-inflammatory medication can be helpful; these may be accessed through your doctor or your employer's occupational health team.

Heavy bleeding/anaemia

Significance/impact: Especially in perimenopause. Symptoms such as unpredictable bleeding, flooding and pelvic pain can affect many work situations and physical distress can occur. If anaemia occurs as a consequence, this can cause lethargy and fatigue and affect productivity at work.

Self-management: Consider discussing treatments to regulate periods with your doctor. Prescription iron supplements may be needed. Ask your employer if you can have some flexibility on the heavy bleeding days if these are predictable. Provision for a shorter working day or working from home on the bad days can help reduce the distress of the symptoms.

Weight gain

Significance/impact: Reduced self-esteem and confidence, which can affect work situations.

Self-management: Monitor and moderate calories. Increase your physical activity if possible. Consider using a fitness app that tracks calories and activity.

NON-MENOPAUSE COEXISTING FACTORS

Your experience of going through menopause in the workplace will be unique and dependent on your work requirements, working hours, work environment, sleep quality, coexisting illnesses, personal and home circumstances, and other external factors that may impact on your symptoms. As a woman going through menopause today you are likely to be part of the 'sandwich generation'; sandwiched between dependent children and elderly parents, which will add another dimension to your busy life.

Carer roles, personal/social/relationship issues

Significance/impact: Demands outside work can impact on your stress, mood, sleep and fatigue. These can all affect work performance.

Self-management: Look at all your commitments and see if there are small changes you can make to improve your quality of life so that you are better able to manage your work requirements and enjoy your job. If you cannot see a solution to outside work commitments and stress then think about work adjustments that would help you continue in work sustainably.

Lifestyle factors

Significance/impact: Smoking, drugs, alcohol misuse, poor diet.

Self-management: Be reflective about whether these are impacting on your work and quality of life. If so, discuss with your doctor what support you can access to help with difficulties.

Additional medical/health problems

Significance/impact: Many separate health issues can be present during menopause and can increase impact on symptoms.

Self-management: Making sure your health issues are all addressed and optimised is important. Other conditions can impact on your menopause symptom burden. Talk to your doctor or practice nurse about whether any treatment adjustments are needed for any additional medical conditions.

A quick recap

Understanding how your menopause symptoms can affect your work will help you to find solutions to them, with the help of your supportive employer. If your employer provides you with reasonable support and adjustments, and makes your workplace menopause-friendly, this will help you to perform to the best of your ability at work.

Breaking down the taboo around menopause in the workplace can be achieved by raising awareness and providing you, where necessary, with supportive work adjustments. These strategies are likely to have benefits for your job satisfaction, morale, motivation and productivity.

CHAPTER 17

A Breast Cancer Journey

WE NEED TO thrive, not just survive. This is the mantra I subscribe to, for living through menopause in general. There is no context to which this is more relevant than women who have also gone through breast cancer and its treatment.

MENOPAUSE NOW

More than 55,000 women are diagnosed with breast cancer every year in the UK. Many will be in menopause and, if they are not, then it may be induced by the treatment they are given. One in eight women will be diagnosed with breast cancer in their lifetime and almost two out of three women with breast cancer now survive their disease beyond twenty years. Survival continues to steadily increase, so breast cancer survivors are a growing demographic among menopausal women.

The majority of chapters in this book are relevant to you even if you cannot safely take hormone therapy, and aim to empower you to understand and take control of your own menopause using self-directed techniques. These can all be applied safely if you are going through breast cancer or if you are a breast cancer survivor. This chapter shares my own experience of breast cancer as a doctor treating it and as a woman going through it and surviving it.

The vast majority of women who have survived breast cancer, in particular hormone-driven breast cancer, will not choose to take HRT as a menopause treatment because of the potential for increasing recurrence risk (see page 190). Hormone receptor-positive breast cancer feeds on oestrogen. It is a deceitful and sly tumour that can lie dormant somewhere in the body until secondary breast cancer appears out of the blue, sometimes even decades later. This happened to Olivia Newton-John after she had been in remission for over 25 years.

Oestrogen-blocking medications, including tamoxifen and aromatase inhibitors, have revolutionised management of breast cancer over the last 30 years and have saved countless lives by suffocating and killing the rogue breast cancer cells that feed on oestrogen. Taking HRT after hormone receptor-positive breast cancer could appear safe for months or years until the recurrence occurs, which may not have happened without oestrogen treatment.

MY CANCER EXPERIENCE

In 1993 when I was a 23-year-old junior doctor, I worked at a world-leading cancer hospital called the Christie Hospital in Manchester. Christie Hospital cancer specialists had done some pioneering work in breast cancer treatment and had been integral in the research trials of the drug tamoxifen. During my junior doctor post as a house officer, I worked on a breast oncology ward and saw many young women being treated in trials of new chemotherapy regimens and tamoxifen to treat their breast cancer. I observed state-of-the-art treatment with new surgical techniques – the so-called wide local excision or lumpectomy surgery – that spared many women from having to have a mastectomy.

It was wonderful to experience how these medical break-throughs could save lives and improve quality of life; my raison d'être as a newly qualified doctor. This has remained a personal purpose for me ever since. At the time, I did not give a single thought to the possibility of going through this myself. I had the protective mindset of denial: 'This will never happen to me!' I loved my job and felt very proud to be working in a world-class hospital that could hopefully find a cure for breast cancer.

But there was also a dark side to that job. As well as seeing new patients going through the journey and accessing amazing new treatments for breast cancer that gave an unprecedented chance of long-term survival, I also saw another story. I saw the women who had received treatment with mastectomy alone, months, years or decades before. If they were found to have cancer in their armpit lymph nodes they may have been offered chemotherapy, but the early regimens were not very successful. Some of these women were returning to the breast cancer club with secondaries. I studied notes thoroughly to find out for myself why these women developed secondary breast cancer. Did they do something wrong? Did they refuse treatment that could have saved them? In all cases the answer was no. Those women had oestrogen-dependent breast cancer and their surgery had not rid them of the so-called 'micro-mets', the rogue cancer cells that can hide for years before returning with a whole cancer army marching unchecked all through the body. Those women had done nothing wrong beyond living in a time that pre-dated effective targeted surgery, chemotherapy, tamoxifen and aromatase inhibitors.

Those beautiful women had their families around them, often young children. No one could do anything to stop that cancer killing them. It was then that I realised a belt-and-braces management approach is best. Playing with breast cancer treatment is like a game of Russian roulette.

Nowadays, things have turned full circle and some of the more recent developments have been to calculate with precision the amount of treatment that is needed. In some cases this means less treatment because the benefits are not outweighed by the risks. Some amazing research progress into early-stage breast cancer can look at genetic characteristics of the tumour to see how likely it is to spread. This helps the breast cancer specialists to identify exactly who needs chemotherapy and other so-called adjuvant treatments and who does not. This is a better way to tackle breast cancer than just 'hoping for the best'. It typifies the dawning of individualised and targeted treatment.

And then I joined the club

On the longest day – 21 June 2011, the summer solstice – I found the lump. It was indeed the longest day for me. I was lucky because my medical knowledge meant I had a pretty good idea of what was coming. The waiting game to find out exactly which branch of the club I was joining was no fun though. Many will relate to that 'no man's land' stage.

I was diagnosed with two early-stage breast cancers simultaneously in one breast. My armpit lymph nodes were clear of cancer but I still wanted belt-and-braces management. I had two young children, a wonderful husband and everything to live for. After my diagnosis, I was told I did not need chemotherapy, even though I was only 41 years old at the time of my diagnosis, i.e. I had premenopausal breast cancer. My cancer was strongly oestrogen receptor-positive. I desperately wanted to be treated with chemotherapy, having seen what had happened to those heroic young women I had cared for at Christie Hospital two decades before. I contacted countless specialists to see if the opinion to withhold chemotherapy was controversial. In fact it became clear to me that the situation had turned full circle. No one recommended chemotherapy and it turned out tamoxifen was going to be my new best friend.

As a hormone specialist I read about the use of chemical menopause for premenopausal women not receiving chemotherapy for breast cancer and the results seemed to be good. So, I persuaded my specialist team to treat me with a chemical menopause – injections that blocked all my hormones. Some of you will have received this treatment. Since my diagnosis this treatment has become more widely used, due to further research showing its benefits, so I feel vindicated in my decision.

I had been interested in menopause since specialising in endocrinology in my twenties, but for the first time, at the age of 42, I truly knew what menopause meant. I broke down in tears in an occupational health meeting that was supposed to be about returning to work (I was mortified because, as my family will testify, I never cry). I then developed horrendous flushes and sweats. I ached all over, I had brain fog and I could not sleep. I knew this all meant I was in menopause with no oestrogen – hooray, I wanted to starve any rogue cancer cells that were trying to sleep in my body, with oestrogen deprivation.

I read Lillie Shockney's inspiring book *Stealing Second Base*, and I would encourage everyone going through breast cancer to read it too. It helped my determination to do all I could to beat my cancer. I watched TV until the small hours, not worrying about lack of sleep, because I knew it didn't really matter. I was fighting that cancer for all the women I had cared for who did not get a second chance. Those women who 'wore my bra before me' did not have the opportunity that I was lucky enough to have; to receive treatment that could statistically result in cure. I gradually made friends with the new me, my body starved of oestrogen (and any rogue cancer cells also starving and perishing, hopefully).

I was initially quite paranoid about every minor symptom I experienced. I do believe that is human nature when you have had a cancer diagnosis, but I gradually learned to mindfully ignore minor symptoms and realised that anything that might need investigating would involve persistent, rather than temporary or fluctuating, symptoms. I mentioned my minor symptoms to one of my wonderful breast cancer team shortly after my treatment completed. She said that I should stop worrying and enjoy the time I have. I have never forgotten those insightful words and I abide by them to this day.

As an endocrinologist, finding myself in a chemical menopause, armed with the knowledge of decades of managing menopause in my patients, I set out to get my life back on track, without HRT of course. I was determined to get well naturally and for the long haul. I was well aware that every woman is individual – no one is average and no one is a statistic. I looked at my own symptoms and tailored management naturally to my own needs. I returned to work four months after my diagnosis. I remember the 'sweat trickling down the back and face' moments, but realised no one else noticed them except me. All the symptoms gradually settled down as I implemented my menopause toolkit and closed each window in my house of menopause. The rest is history. I can honestly say that I feel better now than I felt for most of my premenopausal adult life!

My tips for you

After a breast cancer diagnosis, lifestyle measures are just as important as they are for anyone else going through menopause, but they will also reduce the risk of recurrent or secondary breast cancer, so I could say that the lifestyle toolkit described in Part 2 is even more important if you have had breast cancer.

I am happy to say that this whole book, with the exception of the chapter on HRT, is highly relevant to everyone who is in the breast cancer club. If you can implement some, most or all of the techniques and strategies in the lifestyle toolkit then you will reap the health benefits. You should be able to tailor the techniques to your own personal benefit and needs.

I myself don't have brain fog as long as I do exercise. My feeling is that exercise boosts and regulates my adrenal hormones. The adrenal glands produce sex hormones after menopause and healthy adrenals can, to some extent, make up for the lack of ovarian hormones. This is not a statement based on a research study; it is anecdotal, but it makes logical sense. Exercise does not increase breast cancer risk, it significantly reduces risk. After exercise we also release endorphins that boost our well-being, the so-called happy hormones. If I don't do exercise I feel worse. So I always make time for exercise. I eat healthily and try to moderate alcohol most of the time! I don't believe it is possible to do every-thing perfectly all of the time and no one should beat themselves up about their guilty pleasures – we should enjoy them but we just need to mindfully moderate them.

I use everyday mindfulness techniques for managing stress, but I do not meditate. I tweak as many positive lifestyle changes as I can, but I believe it is impossible to achieve perfection. Small changes are better than no changes. They are also better than a boom-and-bust approach! Trying to follow an unrealistic routine aiming to create perfection is likely to fail.

BREAST CANCER IN YOUNGER WOMEN

About 95 per cent of women diagnosed with breast cancer each year are over the age of 40, and about half are aged 61 and older. Younger women will be more likely to receive chemotherapy or other treatments that cause an early menopause. Keeping heart, blood vessels and bones healthy by using the strategies in my toolkit are particularly important for younger women with treatment-induced early menopause.

> **KEY FACT**
>
> Breast cancer can occur in very young women. Breast cancer in women before the age of 25 is rare, but it can occur, and it should be noted that any woman of any age with concerning breast symptoms should be checked out by a doctor.

Young women may not develop an early menopause through their breast cancer treatment. They may be treated with a chemical menopause, which may be reversible. If you are in this demographic you may have different issues and priorities compared with older women going through breast cancer. For example, you may have young children and/or fertility concerns if you have not had children. It is important to voice any concerns with your cancer teams. You are unlikely to be the first person to ask the question and they are likely to have some answers, be able to signpost you to appropriate resources or refer you to other specialists who can help. This is also true if you are in an ethnic group that culturally does not discuss breast cancer. Support networks and being able to link with people in a similar situation as you can be comforting, inspiring and liberating. These networks are widely available now and your worries and concerns are likely to be lessened if you have this type of support network.

A quick recap

None of us have perfect lives – perfection does not exist! No one chooses breast cancer. It is given to us. Surviving breast cancer is a life challenge that can cause anguish in the short term, but can be enriching in the long term. Grief is a natural feeling after a breast cancer diagnosis because, in some ways, life as you knew it has been lost. Being diagnosed with breast cancer taught me how to appreciate normal life, because that felt like it was gone while I was going through treatment. I appreciated it much more when I got normal life back!

It is important to realise that after breast cancer a new life is beginning. Embracing and focusing on the positive consequences of surviving breast cancer is an important part of acceptance. Thinking about the avenues it opens, and the new life experiences it can generate, will help with acceptance, closure and moving on.

Living Your Best Life

WHEN PEOPLE TALK about menopause there is a tendency to think only of the difficult time when it all begins and short-term coping strategies to get through the challenging phase with teenage kids, demanding employment, care roles and a battery of other unpredictabilities. So, what lies beyond that stage? Perhaps an empty nest, but also less pressure. Senior work roles may gradually carry less onerous and more rewarding commitments, and you may have more time to spend with friends and more time for doing the things you enjoy. Watching your adult children carve out their own lives can be rewarding but also, of course, nail-biting! You are likely to have more time to keep active in ways you enjoy and perhaps additional responsibilities with grandchildren. You may embark on new exciting challenges that you have always desired, but never had the time or opportunity to tackle. You may or may not feel you have more time, depending on what fills your daily routine, but you have the wisdom, knowledge and experience to be the best version of yourself.

You may have decided to continue HRT long-term because it has been a vital crutch for you that you don't want to change. You may have tailed off by now, or never taken it. HRT or not, hopefully you have embraced the lifestyle approaches described in this book, to keep you fit, strong and symptom-free.

If you have exercise engrained in your routine and good approaches to nutrition, sleep and stress management, you will be

MENOPAUSE NOW

There are many more women living a long life after menopause compared with 70 years ago. In 2018, 18 per cent of the total UK population was aged 65 years and over (of whom 55 per cent are women), compared with 10.8 per cent in 1950 – and predicted to be 24.8 per cent in 2050.

in the driving seat living your best life. These provide a blueprint for health and well-being and have the capacity to stave off many illnesses and health issues that can hamper quality of life as time goes on. These simple but amazing lifestyle biohacks are pivotal and can make the difference between lifelong health and premature ageing.

KEY FACT

The average life expectancy in the UK is 82.9 years. Many healthy women will therefore live considerably longer than this.

If you have read this whole book then, whatever your age, you have food for thought about self-empowerment to take control and maintain lifelong health. Investing in lifestyle commitments is investing in your future and will also improve the here-and-now experience; there is no downside.

One of the aims of a successful menopause is to embrace the unpredictability of your individual menopause journey and carve out a path that works for you and leads to a 'third age' of positive attitude, health and vigour (described by historian Peter Laslett in 1987). Your individual path will not be exactly the same as anyone else's. No one else can carve it for you – you are your own menopause expert.

I am often asked whether lifestyle approaches should change as we get older. The short answer is no. The longer answer is that it will depend on the state of your joints, heart and blood vessels, and your overall health. There is a correlation between advancing age and a number of health conditions. If you are an elite athlete, ageing joints may limit some activities and this will be similar in male athletes who are getting older, but you can still maintain exercises that are not traumatic to the joints or likely to induce injuries, such as yoga, Pilates, swimming, cycling and some gym activities. The choice of what you do is down to you. To keep moving remains the perpetual goal.

Maintaining your level of physical fitness during the decades after menopause should be one of your ambitions. Not moving can result in frailty and cause thinning and weakness (disuse atrophy) of all muscles (see page 52). That can increase the risk of falls, resulting in broken bones, which can be serious as we get older.

Other lifestyle approaches do not need to change as you get older; in fact they should get easier as time goes on as your body gets used to implementing them into your routine. We are creatures of habit, so once a routine is established it's easier to maintain.

THE MIND-BODY CONNECTION

Menopause creates tangible, physical, and sometimes very distressing symptoms. Mind-management approaches alone do not reverse underlying problems and are not a panacea, but if you are aware of what to expect, when a symptom appears you will automatically think differently. You will understand the symptom, and you will be more able and motivated to implement appropriate and timely strategies, including mindfulness, that will help your symptoms. Consider the following two scenarios:

Scenario 1: Consider a woman entering menopause. She has developed several physical and psychological symptoms and has no idea what is happening to her body. She starts to think 'My body and mind are falling apart' or 'What is happening to me? This could be really serious', and other thoughts that can be described as catastrophising. In this situation, a woman will have feelings of hopelessness, isolation and fear. The physical fight or flight stress response will be switched on. Negative thoughts can dominate the mind, destructively affecting mood and impacting on relationships, which can have a negative ripple effect on many aspects of the woman's life and the lives of those around her. She may be prescribed medication that does not work or has unpleasant side effects, she may develop worsening sleep issues, and she may use binge eating or drinking alcohol as coping strategies. She is likely to feel exhausted, as anxiety can drain energy. She will then not feel like doing any physical activity. This woman is trapped. This cycle represents a downward spiral of well-being from which it can be difficult to escape.

Scenario 2: Now consider a woman who has been informed about all the symptoms of menopause. Perhaps she has read this book. She understands the importance of lifestyle measures and mindfulness approaches on health and well-being in menopause. She positively implements small lifestyle changes to help with well-being in advance of menopause. She does regular exercise and tries to keep her sleep routine healthy. She eats healthily and ensures she is getting all her micronutrients, including the fish and plant-based essential oils that are good for mood. She has already implemented some stress-management strategies into her busy life that were not very difficult to do. She manages her time carefully and has already targeted and addressed toxic relationships and onerous commitments that she knew were having a negative effect on her stress levels.

Now she starts to notice she is feeling more anxious and realises that her hormones may be causing this as there are no other obvious causes. This woman will realise that the new symptoms she is noticing are related to menopause and are normal, although sometimes tricky and unpleasant to experience.

She tries to take some time out and limits her exposure to situations that might make her anxiety worse, both socially and in the workplace. But she doesn't shut off from the world. She keeps busy and physically active, as she knows these actions will help balance hormone fluctuations and improve sleep quality. Most importantly, she mindfully reflects on the fact that the symptoms are actually normal, they are due to menopause, she is not having a breakdown and she understands the symptoms will pass in time. She notices catastrophising thoughts but doesn't invest in these with her attention or behaviour. She understands that her mind is hardwired to produce these kinds of thoughts, but not becoming aligned with them reduces their impact and the role they play in her life. This woman is liberated and free. She is a menopause success story and she will thrive.

These are two sliding-door scenarios. The difference in starting point is marginal and the difference in outcome is immensely significant. Presence or absence of knowledge, understanding, empowerment and preparation, dovetailed with mindful proactivity and subtle adjustments in many lifestyle and behavioural strategies define the outcome. Some women who are in the informed and prepared second scenario may still need support with hormone or other therapy, but many will not.

SMASHING MENOPAUSE: MAINTAINING WELL-BEING AND HEALTH

Good hydration and nutrition are of paramount importance as we get older, not just for healthy skin but for a healthy mind and body.

Keeping a social network (social capital) is particularly important as we grow older. And I mean face to face. Social media is not a substitute for real-time socialising (at any age), although the latter is more likely to be a positive experience as we get older and in lockdown situations, because it keeps us in touch with a wider family and friends network.

Social interaction facilitates brain stimulation, helps mood and reduces stress. It's been shown that older people are more likely to maintain productive, independent and fulfilling lives if they have access to social capital. Isolation is a dangerous commodity. Older people are especially vulnerable to loneliness and social isolation, and it can have a serious effect on health including low mood and stultification. Social interaction is also likely to stimulate more fun and laughter, and laughter is a stress-reliever and mood-booster. So if you can ensure some laughter in your life it is likely to result in health benefits. Keeping an active social calendar is therefore a must.

Getting enough essential micronutrients through food intake is very important for your skin, hair and nails throughout life, and can make a big difference to how you look and feel as you get older, as well as influencing a number of diseases. You can tend to eat less and make different food choices as you get older. Lower food intake among older people has been associated with lower levels of calcium, iron, zinc, B vitamins and vitamin E. These are all very important micronutrients and keep us healthy. If your diet becomes more limited or is less balanced as you get older, you need to ensure that you get enough of these micronutrients in the food you eat or take a supplement (see Chapter 5).

Smoking, drinking too much alcohol, stress and excessive sun exposure can cause premature ageing, inside and out. It is never too late to stop smoking and it is never too late to address unhealthy drinking habits. Wearing sun protection is no less important as you get older.

Being vigilant about any new health concerns is also more important as you get older. New diseases are more common in older people but most conditions are treatable if detected early and will be less likely to impact on your health and well-being if you seek medical advice without delay.

All these factors can make a positive difference to both how you look and how you feel as you get older. The lifestyle toolkit in this book can help you to stay fit, keep healthy and feel good as the years go by. Making good choices empowers you to control your destiny.

(WHAT'S THE STORY) MENOPAUSE GLORY?

Menopause is a stage of life that should be empowering and liberating. It signifies that you are a mature woman who has built up experience and wisdom. As you pass the physically and psychologically challenging premenopausal phases of your life when there is little head space or time to think, you enter a phase in which you are better able to reflect and you have built up wisdom and maturity that only time can muster. You are better able to rise above minor stresses and you will not 'sweat the small stuff', a nemesis for many younger women today, especially with the added burdens of social media and online life in general. You will be respected and revered by those women. You have a perspective that is invaluable. You are a role model. You are the matriarch. This is a stage in life that should be celebrated.

As a woman going through menopause today you are likely to have more adult life after menopause than you had before it, because we are all living longer. You have the prospect of 15–20 more years in employment. You may be caring for and supporting your young, teenage or adult children. You may be caring for elderly relatives. You may be an equal breadwinner, or the main or sole income generator in the family.

It is vitally important to your loved ones and our whole society for you to remain healthy and strong in the decades after menopause. It is even more important to you as an individual because your quality of life has the potential to be better than at other times in your adult life. You may say that can't be true, but think about the pressures and challenges when you were younger – building a career, relationships, marriage, having kids, financial challenges. Consider the modern pressures of social media and mental health issues escalating in younger people due to the immense pressures of modern life. Quality of life for many premenopausal women is not perfect by any means.

You can inspire those younger women around you so that they want to follow in your footsteps. You are the real deal. You have the power to influence and inspire a generation of young people as they observe your mental and physical strength and resilience. You bring to the world a gift of experience and tenacity. It is a big responsibility because the world needs you. No more menopause muddle. You have read this book, now let's get menopause done and achieve lifelong health.

Frequency of Intake of Certain Foods

Daily essentials

You can have any of these foods on a daily basis depending on your preference. They are all super-nutritious with many health benefits. It is not possible to include every possible option – this list is for guidance only.

- All vegetables and salad leaves; think rainbow colours, e.g. root vegetables, beans, peas, lettuce, peppers, mushrooms, avocados, tomatoes, celery, cucumber, beetroot
- Oats
- Any combination of nuts and seeds
- Any fresh fruit: citrus, berry, tropical
- Dried fruit
- Hummus
- Soy products
- Tofu
- Brown rice
- Eggs
- Lentils, beans, peas, chickpeas
- Wholegrain cereals
- Low-fat dairy or non-dairy alternative
- Wholemeal or sourdough bread

- Fermented foods, e.g. tempeh, miso, kimchi, sauerkraut, kefir, kombucha, live yoghurt
- Plenty of water to keep hydrated. Tea and coffee can be taken daily but try to limit to two or three cups per day and avoid caffeine in the evening close to bedtime

Less than daily

These foods will provide more nutrients but are not needed daily. They can be alternated on different days depending on your dietary preference.

- White meat
- Oily fish
- Shellfish
- River fish

Once or twice per week

Try to limit these foods to once or twice per week.

- Organ meats
- Red meat
- Full-fat dairy (cheese, chocolate, cream, full-cream milk)
- Fruit juices (these often contain vitamin C but can be very high in sugar and do not have the fibre that is present in the whole fruit)

Non-essential

These foods are not essential and should be limited where possible.

- White bread, white pasta, shop-bought cakes, biscuits, pizza, pastries (if you eat foods from the lists above you will be getting enough slow-release carbs and so these rapid-release processed carbs may lead to bloating and weight gain)

- Processed, smoked and cured meats
- Processed ready meals
- Coffee-shop-bought cappuccinos and other high-calorie drinks
- Fizzy drinks

Other considerations

Alcohol

If you like to drink alcohol, try to limit your intake to 14 units per week and have 2 or 3 alcohol-free days during the week. Remember there are a lot of calories in the form of sugar in alcohol with no nutrients (Guinness actually contains very little iron!).

Salt

Try to use iodised salt when cooking from scratch. Stock cubes contain quite a lot of salt. Processed foods already have a lot of salt added, so if you do eat processed food try not to use any added salt. Remember too much salt can cause high blood pressure.

Portion sizes

The portion sizes that you need to keep a steady weight will depend on your level of activity and your metabolism. We know that there are genetic factors contributing to weight, so in menopause some women will get away with eating larger portions than others, depending on these factors. However, you should always be mindful of eating healthily.

Your meals should provide an optimal amount of protein, fibre and micronutrients. The total calories will depend on your portion sizes and your consumption of guilty pleasures.

Sample Weekly Menu

THIS MENU IS an example of foods that can mostly be cooked from scratch and provide lots of micronutrients and fibre, adequate protein and low refined sugar or processed ingredients. It is flexitarian and can easily be adapted to be vegetarian or vegan. It is for general guidance only. If you are not burning many calories then you may need to cut the desserts out on several days per week. Portion sizes will depend on your activity and calories burned.

Snacks: Almonds, cashew or peanuts, dried fruit/fresh fruit, vegetable sticks with hummus or cottage cheese, olives, edamame beans, air-popped popcorn. Try kombucha. Portions will depend on your activity and level of calorie-burning.

You can, of course, add your guilty pleasures here and there, but consumption of these needs to be sparing to keep your weight steady.

Meal	Monday	Tuesday	Wednesday	Thursday	Friday	Saturday	Sunday
Breakfast	Porridge (add berries/fruit/flaxseeds to taste)	High-protein bagel with smoked salmon and cream cheese	Wholegrain cereal with kefir yoghurt or almond milk	Fruit smoothie with chia seeds or sardines on toast	Porridge with chia seeds and dried fruit	Baked beans/eggs with mushrooms on wholemeal toast	Eggs/spinach on sourdough toast
Lunch	Butternut squash risotto with sourdough bread	Vegetable and lentil soup Flapjack	Hummus or mackerel pâté, pitta bread, salad and sauerkraut Fresh fruit	Quinoa salad Fruit cake	Spinach and tomato omelette Fresh fruit	Wholemeal pasta with tomato/pesto sauce	Jacket potato with tuna/cottage cheese and salad
Dinner	Lean meat/salmon/tofu with roasted vegetables and brown rice or potatoes with skin on Optional: ice cream/sorbet	Chickpea and spinach curry, lentil dhal and roasted cauliflower Optional: rice pudding	Vegetarian or meat chilli con carne, extra red kidney beans Optional: baked banana with kirsch and yoghurt	Chicken/fish/vegetable paella Optional: summer fruit compote	Stir-fried steak/tofu/chicken/veg with bean sprouts and kimchi Optional: home-made cake/fresh berries	Chicken/veg and coconut curry with egg- or spinach-fried rice Optional: baked apple and kefir yoghurt	Nut roast or roast dinner Optional: cheese/grapes
Time-restricted	Try to do time-restricted eating (window of 8–12 hours for all your food intake – see page 114) for 3–5 days out of 7.						

Macronutrient Balance

Fibre: Aim for 20–30g daily

Food source examples	Grams of fibre (approximate)
Almonds (1 handful; 28g)	3.5
Apple (1)	4.4
Avocado (1)	13
Banana (1)	3
Beetroot (136g)	2.8
Broccoli (91g)	2.3
Brussels sprouts (100g)	2.6
Carrots (100g)	2.8
Cauliflower (150g)	3.8
Chia seeds (28g)	11
Chickpeas (120g)	8.3
Dark chocolate >70% cocoa solids (28g)	2.3
Dried apricots/dates/prunes (100g)	7
Hummus (100g)	6
Kidney beans (50g)	12.5
Lentils (100g)	8
Oats (100g)	10.1
Peanuts (50g)	4.3
Pear (1 medium)	5.5
Potato, with skin (1 medium)	4
Quinoa (100g)	10

Raspberries (100g)	7
Sourdough or wholemeal bread (1 slice)	2
Spinach, cooked (100g)	2.2
Strawberries (100g)	2
Sweet potato, no skin (1 medium)	3.8
Wholemeal bagel (1)	7

Protein: Aim for around 50g daily

Food source examples	Grams of protein (approximate)
Almonds (1 handful; 28g)	6
Beef steak (100g)	26
Broccoli (100g)	2.8
Chicken breast, no skin (100g)	26
Chickpeas (1 x 120-g tin)	8.1
Egg (1)	6
Hummus (100g)	7.9
Lentils (100g)	9
Milk (250ml)	8
Oats (100g)	10.3
Peanuts (50g)	15
Pitta bread (1 large)	6
Pork (85g)	23
Prawns (85)	12
Pumpkin/sunflower/chia seeds (28g)	4
Quinoa (100g)	4.4
Red kidney beans (1 x 200-g tin)	10
Salmon (85g)	18.3
Tofu (150g)	8
Tuna (two-thirds of a 145-g tin)	27
Turkey breast (85g)	26
Wholemeal bagel (1)	11
Wholemeal bread (1 slice)	2.5
Yoghurt (100g)	3.5

References

CHAPTER 2: DEMYSTIFYING SYMPTOMS

Baker, C. (6 Aug. 2019). House of Commons library briefing paper number 3336. Obesity statistics.

Prague, J. K., Roberts, R. E., Comninos, A. N., Clarke, S., Jayasena, C. N., Nash, Z., Doyle, C., Papadopoulou, D. A., Bloom, S. R., Mohideen, P. and Panay, N., 2017. Neurokinin 3 receptor antagonism as a novel treatment for menopausal hot flushes: A phase 2, randomised, double-blind, placebo-controlled trial. *The Lancet*, *389*(10081), pp. 1775–7.

CHAPTER 5: AN A TO Z OF NUTRIENTS IN MENOPAUSE

Makki, K., Deehan, E. C., Walter, J. and Bäckhed, F., 2018. The impact of dietary fiber on gut microbiota in host health and disease. *Cell Host & Microbe*, *23*(6), pp. 705–15.

CHAPTER 6: FIGHTING FLUSHES AND SWEATS

Carpenter, J., Gass, M. L., Maki, P. M., Newton, K. M., Pinkerton, J. V., Taylor, M., Utian, W. H., Schnatz, P. F., Kaunitz, A. M., Shapiro, M. and Shifren, J. L., 2015. Nonhormonal management of menopause-associated vasomotor symptoms: 2015 position statement of The North American Menopause Society. *Menopause*, *22*(11), pp. 1155–72.

Fenlon, D., Nuttall, J., May, C., Raftery, J., Fields, J., Kirkpatrick, E., Abab, J., Ellis, M., Rose, T., Khambhaita, P. and Galanopoulou, A., 2018. MENOS4 trial: A multicentre randomised controlled trial (RCT) of a breast care nurse delivered cognitive behavioural therapy (CBT) intervention to reduce the impact of hot flushes in women with breast cancer: Study Protocol. *BMC Women's Health*, 18(1), p. 63.

CHAPTER 7: MANAGING YOUR SLEEP

Harvard Health Letter (13 Aug. 2018). Blue light has a dark side. Retrieved from https://www.health.harvard.edu/staying-healthy/blue-light-has-a-dark-side.

Kervezee, L., Kosmadopoulos, A. and Boivin, D. B., 2020. Metabolic and cardiovascular consequences of shift work: The role of circadian disruption and sleep disturbances. *European Journal of Neuroscience*, 51(1), pp. 396–412.

Wang, C., Bangdiwala, S. I., Rangarajan, S., Lear, S. A., AlHabib, K. F., Mohan, V., Teo, K., Poirier, P., Tse, L. A., Liu, Z. and Rosengren, A., 2019. Association of estimated sleep duration and naps with mortality and cardiovascular events: A study of 116, 632 people from 21 countries. *European Heart Journal*, 40(20), pp. 1620–9.

CHAPTER 8: WEIGHT MANAGEMENT

Afzal, S., Tybjærg-Hansen, A., Jensen, G. B. and Nordestgaard, B. G., 2016. Change in body mass index associated with lowest mortality in Denmark, 1976–2013. *JAMA*, 315(18), pp. 1989–96.

Gabel, K., Hoddy, K. K., Haggerty, N., Song, J., Kroeger, C. M., Trepanowski, J. F., Panda, S. and Varady, K. A., 2018. Effects of 8-hour time restricted feeding on body weight and metabolic disease risk factors in obese adults: A pilot study. *Nutrition and Healthy Aging*, 4(4), pp. 345–53.

CHAPTER 9: UNDERSTANDING STRESS

McEwen, B. S., 2005. Stressed or stressed out: What is the difference? *Journal of Psychiatry and Neuroscience*, *30*(5), pp. 315–8.

McEwen, B. S. and Stellar, E., 1993. Stress and the individual: Mechanisms leading to disease. *Archives of Internal Medicine*, *153*(18), pp. 2093–101.

CHAPTER 12: BONE HEALTH

Weaver, C. M., Gordon, C. M., Janz, K. F., Kalkwarf, H. J., Lappe, J. M., Lewis, R., O'Karma, M., Wallace, T. C. and Zemel, B. S., 2016. The National Osteoporosis Foundation's position statement on peak bone mass development and lifestyle factors: A systematic review and implementation recommendations. *Osteoporosis International*, *27*(4), pp. 1281–386.

CHAPTER 13: NATURAL AND COMPLEMENTARY REMEDIES

Booth, N. L., Piersen, C. E., Banuvar, S., Geller, S. E., Shulman, L. P. and Farnsworth, N. R., 2006. Clinical studies of red clover (Trifolium pratense) dietary supplements in menopause: A literature review. *Menopause*, *13*(2), pp. 251–64.

Hirata, J. D., Swiersz, L. M., Zell, B., Small, R. and Ettinger, B., 1997. Does dong quai have estrogenic effects in postmenopausal women? A double-blind, placebo-controlled trial. *Fertility and Sterility*, *68*(6), pp. 981–6.

Kargozar, R., Azizi, H. and Salari, R., 2017. A review of effective herbal medicines in controlling menopausal symptoms. *Electronic Physician*, *9*(11), pp. 5826–33.

Kim, M. S., Lim, H. J., Yang, H. J., Lee, M. S., Shin, B. C. and Ernst, E., 2013. Ginseng for managing menopause symptoms: A systematic review of randomized clinical trials. *Journal of Ginseng Research*, 37(1), pp. 30–6.

Leach, M. J. and Moore, V., 2012. Black cohosh (Cimicifuga spp.) for menopausal symptoms. *Cochrane Database of Systematic Reviews*, (9), CD007244.

Linde, K., Berner, M. M. and Kriston, L., 2008. St John's wort for major depression. *Cochrane Database of Systematic Reviews*, (4), CD000448.

Wuttke, W., Jarry, H., Haunschild, J., Stecher, G., Schuh, M. and Seidlova-Wuttke, D., 2014. The non-estrogenic alternative for the treatment of climacteric complaints: Black cohosh (Cimicifuga or Actaea racemosa). *The Journal of Steroid Biochemistry and Molecular Biology*, 139, pp. 302–10.

CHAPTER 14: SEX AND INTIMACY

Dizavandi, F. R., Ghazanfarpour, M., Roozbeh, N., Kargarfard, L., Khadivzadeh, T. and Dashti, S., 2019. An overview of the phytoestrogen effect on vaginal health and dyspareunia in peri-and postmenopausal women. *Post Reproductive Health*, 25(1), pp. 11–20.

Knight, C., Logan, V. and Fenlon, D., 2019. A systematic review of laser therapy for vulvovaginal atrophy/genitourinary syndrome of menopause in breast cancer survivors. *ecancer*, 13, 988.

Melisko, M. E., Goldman, M. E., Hwang, J., De Luca, A., Fang, S., Esserman, L. J., Chien, A. J., Park, J. W. and Rugo, H. S., 2017. Vaginal testosterone cream vs estradiol vaginal ring for vaginal dryness or decreased libido in women receiving aromatase inhibitors for early-stage breast cancer: A randomized clinical trial. *JAMA Oncology*, 3(3), pp. 313–9.

Pickar, J. H., Boucher, M. and Morgenstern, D., 2018. Tissue selective estrogen complex (TSEC): A review. *Menopause*, 25(9), pp. 1033–45.

CHAPTER 15: HORMONE REPLACEMENT THERAPY (HRT)

Collaborative Group on Hormonal Factors in Breast Cancer, 2019. Type and timing of menopausal hormone therapy and breast cancer risk: Individual participant meta-analysis of the worldwide epidemiological evidence. *The Lancet*, 394(10204), pp. 1113–204.

Mirkin, S., 2018. Evidence on the use of progesterone in menopausal hormone therapy. *Climacteric*, 21(4), pp. 346–54.

Newson, L. and Rymer, J., 2019. The dangers of compounded bioidentical hormone replacement therapy. *British Journal of General Practice*, 69(688), pp. 540–1.

NICE (2019). Summary of evidence for 2019 surveillance of menopause (2015) NICE guideline NG23. Retrieved from https://www.nice.org.uk/consultations/672/10/long-term-benefits-and-risks-of-hormone-replacement-therapy.

CHAPTER 16: MENOPAUSE AT WORK

CIPD (26 Mar. 2019). The menopause at work: Guidance for people professionals. Retrieved from https://www.cipd.co.uk/knowledge/culture/well-being/menopause/people-professionals-guidance?utm_source=google&utm_medium=cpc&utm_campaign=menopauseatwork&utm_content=MAW_PPC_BMM&gclid=Cj0KCQjwpLfzBRCRARIsAHuj6qWKm1oxBI1WZdLjBV_yMEnZTwZgHo3AeirthNkG8gA664zeNfcWJpwaApj-YEALw_wcB.

Faculty of Occupational Medicine. Health and work: Menopause focus. Retrieved from http://www.fom.ac.uk/wp-content/uploads/Menopause-Focus-Infographic.pdf.

Hardy, C., Griffiths, A., Thorne, E. and Hunter, M. S., 2019. Tackling the taboo: Talking menopause-related problems at work. *International Journal of Workplace Health Management*, 12(1), pp. 28–38.

Hardy, C., Thorne, E., Griffiths, A. and Hunter, M. S., 2018. Work outcomes in midlife women: The impact of menopause, work stress and working environment. *Women's Midlife Health*, 4(1), p. 3.

Office for National Statistics (16 Jul. 2019). Employment in the UK: July 2019. Retrieved from https://www.ons.gov.uk/employment-andlabourmarket/peopleinwork/employmentandemployeetypes/bulletins/employmentintheuk/july2019.

CONCLUSION: LIVING YOUR BEST LIFE

Office for National Statistics. Living longer: Is age 70 the new age 65? Retrieved from https://www.ons.gov.uk/peoplepopula-tionandcommunity/birthsdeathsandmarriages/ageing/articles/livinglongerisage70thenewage65/2019–11-19.

Office for National Statistics (25 Sep. 2019). National life tables, UK: 2016 to 2018. Retrieved from https://www.ons.gov.uk/peoplepopulationandcommunity/birthsdeathsandmarriages/lifeexpectancies/bulletins/nationallifetablesunitedkingdom/2016to2018.

INDEX

AM indicates Dr Annice Mukherjee
Page references in *italics* indicate images.